WRONGFUL ACTS

TONY SCLAMA

Tony Sclama

Tony Sclama Books

First paperback edition 2021

Published by Tony Sclama Books

www.tonysclama.com

Cover and Interior Design by Ebook Launch

ISBN 978-1-7372656-0-3

Library of Congress Control Number: 2021911120

CHAPTER

ONE

"Dan? Dan! Are you listening to me?"

Paul Bellini and his lifelong friend, Dan Cliffden, were in the middle of a conversation over dinner while their wives chatted across the table.

Cliffden had suddenly stopped responding, looking at his friend with a blank stare.

The waitress came over holding a tray with the two beers Bellini had ordered for them.

"What's the matter with your friend? He looks like he just saw a ghost."

Bellini shrugged. "Dunno. He just stopped talking, and that blank stare hasn't changed since. Hasn't moved either, or as much as blinked."

He reached out to his friend and lightly touched his wrist to shake it. "Are you okay, Dan? Is something wrong? Come on, guy. Talk to me."

Nothing. Only that blank stare.

Having noticed what was transpiring between their husbands, the two wives stopped talking and looked over.

Without any warning, Cliffden leaned over the table and forcefully grabbed Bellini around his neck with both hands.

The waitress gasped as she stepped back, the tray and beers crashing to the floor.

"What...the...hell," grunted Bellini, barely audible.

He reached up to pull Cliffden's hands away, but the grip just tightened.

Cliffden's wife stood and grabbed him by the shoulders. "Stop, Dan! Stop!" she yelled. "What are you doing?"

It had no effect.

Bellini felt a crushing sensation in his throat and couldn't breathe. The throbbing pressure in his head made him feel like it was about to explode, and his vision blurred. Unable to get air, the burning in his chest was unbearable.

A diner from a nearby table came over and yelled at Cliffden. "What the hell are you doin, man? You're gonna kill him." Bellini now had a bluish tinge to his face and the stranger tried to pull Cliffden's hands away from Bellini, but he couldn't break the grip.

More people gathered. The bartender came over to help but likewise failed.

Bellini felt the room spinning. His head in a fog, he reached for the table to steady himself. As he moved his hands over the surface, he felt something cold. *A knife.* He picked it up and with the little strength he had left plunged the blade deep into the neck of his best friend.

CHAPTER

TWO

"Have a seat," said Constance Vasquez, standing in front of a bookcase.

Dr. Allisyn McLoren was fifteen minutes early for her meeting with the Secretary of Health and Human Services in the Hubert H. Humphrey Building in Southwest D.C. As commissioner of the Food and Drug Administration, Allisyn reported directly to the HHS Secretary. In her role as head of the FDA, she provided operational, policy and regulatory oversight of the federal agency which is tasked with evaluating and approving all human therapeutic drugs, biologic products and medical devices.

A physician with a PhD in genetics and a Nobel Prize for her genomics research, Allisyn was chosen to lead the FDA to correct the numerous deficiencies which had plagued the agency for several years and were the subject of severe criticism.

Now, after having recently completed her second year in the role, she took pride in successfully rehabilitating the troubled agency and restoring confidence in the execution of its mission. Despite her success, however, Allisyn dreaded her meetings with the secretary.

Vasquez was not a physician. In fact, her only health care experience had been as CEO of a major health insurance company. She related to every issue from a rigid business perspective, often with a political bias. As a result, Allisyn always approached their discussions with a healthy dose of skepticism.

Even though she had a world-renowned reputation as a re-search scientist, Allisyn knew the role of commissioner would be challenging enough given the troubled FDA's recently blemished history. And the politically charged Washington environment added fuel to the fire. What she didn't anticipate, however—and certainly did not need—was an overbearing boss.

As Vasquez walked around the desk and sat in her chair, Al-lisyn questioned her choice of clothes for the day. Knee-length wool skirt, print blouse and navy blue cardigan. The secretary was more formally attired in a classic woman's business suit. Gray tweed blazer over a beige blouse and black silk slacks.

Oh well, Allisyn thought as she took a seat at one of the side chairs opposite Vasquez. She wondered why they weren't using the more comfortable armchairs across the room as they usually did for their informal meetings. Looking around, she thought how remarkably different the secretary's elaborate office decor was from her own minimalist style.

"Thanks for agreeing to this last-minute meeting," said Vasquez. "I've been really busy and time got away from me. I wanted to touch base with you regarding the upcoming congres-sional hearing and your prepared comments."

Allisyn was to testify in front of a Senate subcommittee re-garding the status of the changes made at the FDA.

"No problem. Always happy to keep you updated. Anything specific?"

"Now I know this is your report, Allisyn, not mine." She leaned forward with hands folded and elbows on the desk. "From the beginning of your tenure, however, expectations have been extremely high for restoring the agency's reputation. I simply have a few questions to make sure we're on the same page."

"Sure. Fire away." Despite her response, Allisyn was suspect about where this was going.

"I presume you'll focus on the changes you've made. Correct?"

"Of course. I imagine it's what the committee members expect."

"Anything in particular?"

"For starters, I'm sure the senators will want to hear what we've done to prevent the inappropriate influence the pharmaceutical industry and their lobbyists were previously exerting on the FDA."

"Mm-hmm. And what about the issue of regulatory inconsistency?"

A little odd, thought Allisyn when Vasquez changed the subject. "I'm confident we've adequately addressed those concerns as well."

Vasquez frowned. "I'm well aware of your position on underregulation and inadequate oversight of the review process. But what about the issue of overregulation?"

Allisyn hesitated, folding her arms and tilting her head. "What about it?"

"Well, everyone knows overregulation has been blamed for excessive delays in the drug approval process."

"True, but inadequate oversight can result in problems much more serious than delays. Safety should always be our first priority."

Vasquez leaned back in her chair. "Of course, of course. I'm not implying otherwise, Allisyn. However, it's important we reassure our constituents they'll have access to new and innovative treatments in a timely fashion."

Allisyn shifted in her chair and remained tight-lipped.

Vasquez broke the awkward silence. "Okay, then. I'm sure our colleagues on the hill will indeed be pleased with the results of your efforts to turn the agency around in a positive direction."

Allisyn suddenly felt uncomfortable. *I gotta get outta here as quickly as possible.* "Unless you have anything else, I should be going. The rest of my day is packed and I'm sure you have a busy day ahead as well." She placed her hands on the arms of the chair to push herself up.

Vasquez leaned forward. "Remember, Allisyn, don't over-emphasize the need for tight control on the review process."

Allisyn's back stiffened as she proceeded to stand.

The secretary remained seated. "After all, it's imperative the committee and the public have full confidence in the commitment of the FDA to approve cutting edge therapies in a timely fashion. And that is especially true of the agency's commissioner."

Allisyn felt her stomach churn and didn't respond.

Vasquez abruptly stood herself and stared directly at her. "I think we're good to go, then."

"See you at the hearing," Allisyn said, half looking back over her shoulder as she left.

On the return trip to her office, she thought about how uncomfortable the meeting had been. Especially the secretary's unsettling directive.

Strange. Very strange.

The remainder of Allisyn's day consisted of a series of meetings, and she didn't return to her office at the FDA until late afternoon. When she arrived, she was greeted by her assistant, Ginger, who dutifully followed her with a cup of coffee, placed it on the desk in front of the commissioner and sat across from her.

"Here's the notes you wanted for your upcoming report, Allisyn" said Ginger, handing her a Manila folder.

From the beginning of her tenure, Allisyn encouraged an informal working relationship with her assistant, and it had worked out well so far.

"Thanks. I'll review them at home." Allisyn placed the folder on her desktop among the many other papers and folders already scattered over it.

"How did your meeting with the secretary go?"

Allisyn rolled her eyes. "Don't even mention it."

"As usual, eh?"

Allisyn only nodded.

Ginger glanced at the clock on the credenza behind Allisyn below her framed medical degree and award citation from the Norwegian Nobel Committee.

"Oh my gosh! It's after six," said Ginger as she pushed forward in her chair. "I gotta go. Give me a call if you have any questions."

"Will do."

When she heard the office suite door close, Allisyn sighed, leaned back in her chair, kicked off her heels and placed her legs on the desk, her slender ankles crossed. Thinking of Secretary Vasquez's office décor, she looked around her office and wondered if she should dress it up some. There were shelves of professional texts and journals and several filing cabinets matching her desk but few personal items save for the various framed certificates and credentials on the walls. *Perhaps some flowers? No way. Plants? Maybe.* This was an exercise she performed periodically, each time reaching the same conclusion. *The office is fine the way it is.*

She opened the folder and rifled through the pages, conversant with all the relevant issues she wanted to address at her upcoming report to the Congressional Oversight Committee. She would be reporting to the members on the status of her work in restoring legitimacy to the previously mismanaged agency. After about ten minutes, she decided to finish later. She stood and slipped into her shoes, placed the folder in her briefcase with some other papers and headed home.

CHAPTER

THREE

"I would like to call this meeting to order," said the committee chair.

Senator Carlton Gradison banged the gavel to convene the day's meeting of the Senate Committee on Health, Education, Labor and Pensions—HELP. The HELP Committee provided congressional oversight for most of the HHS agencies, including the FDA. Allisyn was about to testify in this same chamber of the Dirksen Senate Office Building where her confirmation hearings were held.

Before taking her seat at the guest table, she scanned the gallery behind her. It was filled with staffers, members of the media and other interested parties, including Constance Vasquez. When their eyes met, the secretary remained impassive as Allisyn acknowledged her presence by nodding.

"I'd like to welcome everyone to today's proceedings," said Gradison once the pre-meeting chatter in the room quieted. "And a special welcome to Commissioner McLoren for joining us today."

He offered some complimentary remarks regarding improvements made at the FDA under her leadership before giving her the floor to provide her report. Questions from committee members would follow.

"Thank you for such a kind introduction, Mr. Chairman." Allisyn scanned the committee membership sitting at the tiered seating in front of her. Her immediate impression was her comments were anxiously anticipated.

"Let me start," said Gradison, "by asking you to address some of the concerns we've had about the FDA's previous performance."

Allisyn cleared her throat. "Certainly, Senator. To start, I would like to reassure the committee and the public we are committed to protecting them in the important task of ensuring both the effectiveness and safety of all the various medications, treatments, devices and related products coming before us for review and potential approval. We are also concerned with the safety of those individuals who participate in the clinical trials supporting all proposed new treatments."

"Could you tell us a little about the specific reforms you've made along those lines?" asked Gradison.

"Of course. We've implemented protocol changes in the oversight of how new therapies and products are evaluated. This starts with a strict, non-biased approach on the part of our application review teams."

"Could you elaborate, Doctor?"

Allisyn took a small sip of water. "As we all know, the agency had serious problems around inappropriate industry bias and data mismanagement. This included its failure to consistently identify fraudulent research data and report the details of such misconduct to the appropriate parties. In fact, you may recall a group of FDA scientists themselves had raised concerns of pressure from management to manipulate data in new therapy applications."

She paused to gauge the panel's reaction to her opening statement so far and didn't appreciate anything notable.

"Our revised policies and protocols are designed to guard against and prevent those specific issues. I refer you to the technical details which are delineated more thoroughly in my written report,"

Gradison approached the microphone and leaned his folded arms on the desk. "Policies and protocols are wonderful tools, Commissioner, but we all know they must be strictly followed if they're going to be effective. How can you assure this committee and the public adherence to policy is happening and these measures are actually working the way you expected?"

"Great question, Senator. Periodic internal and external audits are utilized to ensure these processes are strictly and consistently followed in a non-biased fashion and are achieving the desired outcome."

"And what do those audits show?"

"To date, we're running at ninety-nine percent compliance. The audits have shown the one-percent outliers relate to minor administrative documentation errors and not technical or data management issues. When identified, such errors are corrected and follow-up audits are performed to ensure they do not recur. So far, none of this small sample of errors relative to the number of applications we review have affected the efficacy of our assessment of the therapy involved."

"Quite impressive, Doctor." Gradison paused, looking down at some notes. "I would like to switch gears and have you address the issue of making new treatments available to patients in a timely fashion. I'm sure you know the public has expressed concerns about delays in beneficial treatments reaching the market. And this committee has pledged to ensure our constituents such unnecessary delays are prevented."

Allisyn recalled her conversation with Constance Vasquez and could almost hear her saying, "Told you so!"

"As we here at the FDA are as well," said Allisyn in response to Gradison's comment. "I assume you're speaking about previous complaints of overregulation. In response to those concerns, we've redesigned our processes to eliminate unnecessary delays in evaluating new therapeutic products. Our goal is to minimize the risk of delays in market availability of approved products.

However, allow me to add a caveat to that objective. The opposite problem of underregulation poses a potentially greater risk. Shortcuts to rush the evaluation process can lead to significant safety issues if complications of a treatment are not identified and addressed prior to market. We cannot sacrifice safety for the expediency of availability."

Appearing satisfied, Gradison asked one more question. "Can you speak to how all these changes have been accepted by your staff?"

Allisyn beamed. "I'm glad you asked that question, Senator. As a side benefit of all this work, we have seen staff productivity and satisfaction increase dramatically. And recent surveys of consumers, health professionals, patients and industry representatives have shown an equally dramatic increase in the trust they place in the agency's decisions. As an example, at a favorable rating of over eighty percent, the FDA far exceeds approval for government agencies in general."

Her last comment was met with laughter throughout the chamber. It even drew smiles from several committee members, including the chair himself.

"Nicely done, Doctor," said Gradison when the stirring simmered down. "Thank you for an excellent summary. I urge the committee members to review your written comments which contain further details on all these issues." He paused. "Before opening the floor for questions, do you have any other remarks?"

"Yes. I'd like to briefly address the topic of gene therapy. I know the committee shares the public's interest in the potential of this new form of therapy."

"Wonderful, Doctor. Please proceed."

She paused to take another short sip of water. "The complex nature of genomics and this form of therapy, along with the numerous ongoing studies seeking product approval for market access, make this one of our more exciting, albeit challenging, endeavors. Changing the genetic makeup of diseased cells holds the potential to treat certain genetically caused diseases which are otherwise untreatable or currently sub-optimally treated. Although genomic research is not new, however, gene therapy as a routine modality of medical treatment is still in its developmental stage.

"The Center for Biologics Evaluation and Research—CBER—is the agency's division overseeing all clinical trials using our standard protocols to ensure efficacy and safety. Gene therapy trials are no different and are subject to the same rigorous scrutiny. Because gene therapy technology actually alters the DNA of one's cells, however, the evaluation of the short- and long-term effects are somewhat more complicated than more traditional forms of therapy.

"And although gene therapy research and development continue to grow at a rapid pace, it still remains available primarily in a research setting. A number of final phase three human clinical trials are currently ongoing, but only a very small number of such treatments have been approved for general use. This is because of the uncertainty of potential side effects from the viral delivery of the therapy. However, CBER is currently reviewing one particular application for a novel form of gene therapy which does not utilize a virus delivery system. We will certainly keep the committee updated as therapies are approved for market access."

She concluded her report by thanking the committee for their attention and offered to answer any questions.

Senator Gradison and several other members offered complimentary remarks regarding her success in rehabilitating the FDA and restoring confidence in its work. Only one other senator had a question. And he had a different agenda.

Senator Winston Lancaster III of Mississippi was known for being blustery and cantankerous and had become more so in the last few years. His heavy Southern drawl was unmistakable.

"Thank you for the report, Doctor. Now I appreciate your assurances about the FDA's intention to protect itself from industry bias, but I've a question about bias within the agency itself." He paused and shuffled through some papers. "Is it fair to say you're the expert in the field of gene research?"

"I don't really know about 'the' expert, but I do have a good bit of experience, yes." A few muffled comments were audible.

"Come now, Doctor. No need to be modest. Didn't you receive some, uh, special recognition? Some award…or somethin'?"

Allisyn struggled to keep a straight face. "Yes, something along those lines."

Now, there were clearly audible chuckles throughout the room.

Could the befuddled Senator be the only one present who doesn't know or possibly forgot I was corecipient of the Nobel Prize four years ago?

Apparently, the befuddled Senator didn't recall that—thirty-four at the time—she was the youngest female to receive the coveted award for Science or Medicine, besting Marie Curie by a couple of years.

Lancaster was unfazed by the gallery's reaction. "And before you assumed your current position with the FDA, you spent a good number of years doin' gene research. Ain't that right?"

"Yes."

"Then I would think you have a vested interest in seein' gene research advance beyond experiments and become a marketable product. A fair assumption, Doctor?"

Allisyn hesitated and shifted slightly in her seat. "I believe everyone would agree if there's a safe and effective scientific discovery which could treat illnesses for which other treatments have been less successful, it would be a scientific advance for all and not solely a success for any one individual." She paused, wondering if she should continue. *Why not?* "After all, I don't think Fleming really had personal accolades or profit in mind while doing his work."

"Ah yes. Sir Ian Fleming," said Lancaster smugly.

Some muted "Huh's" could be heard throughout the room.

"No." She paused and placed a folded hand over her mouth, took several short deliberate breaths, then placed her hand back on the table. "That would be Alexander Fleming. He discovered penicillin."

The chuckles were now louder and more numerous.

Allisyn was starting to feel embarrassed for the Senator and struggled to keep a smile from crossing her lips.

Lancaster ignored her comment and cleared his throat. "Is it not customary for experienced researchers to have a financial interest in their research, Doctor?"

"Like any other gainful employment, I would say most researchers are compensated for the work they do." *Bad girl,* thought Allisyn while biting her lower lip.

"I'm not talkin' 'bout a salary, Doctor," bellowed the Senator. "Can experienced researchers have a financial investment in their research? Ya know, profit from sales?"

Allisyn quickly composed herself. "In certain instances, yes. But such arrangements are not illegal in and of themselves as long as there is nothing untoward about the actual research and their data is factual and valid. The FDA now has strong guidelines and disclosure policies to uncover those situations and ensure data integrity,"

The Senator leaned forward, his eyes intently focused on Allisyn, hands flat on his table.

Allisyn facetiously thought it looked as if he was going to jump out of his seat toward her.

His voice bellowed, "And Doctor, do you—"

"Senator, if you're going to ask whether I or anyone in the agency has such a financial interest in any of the gene therapy products under investigational review or other products we regulate, the answer is categorically no. I personally have no investments or financial interests relative to any of the research I've been involved with or is currently under review. I can reassure the committee there are adequate safeguards within our processes to prevent any internal agency bias to approve research which does not substantiate the proposed outcomes or support approval of the product."

Lancaster seemed at a loss for words. He fell back in his chair, looking down again and shuffling some papers haphazardly. Without looking up, he grumbled, "I yield back, Mr. Chairman."

Gradison quickly took the opportunity to adjourn the session and thanked Allisyn for her time and expertise.

She gathered her notes and headed towards the exit. Constance Vasquez approached Allisyn with a scowl on her face, passing by without stopping.

CHAPTER

FOUR

Carlton Gradison sat at his desk in the Russell Senate Office Building. Located on Constitution Avenue across from the Capitol, the building is the oldest of the three Senate buildings. Although rising five stories above ground on the side opposite the Capitol, the steep slope of the side streets results in only three stories above ground on the Capitol side. This architectural accommodation was intentional to conform to the scale of the Capitol building itself.

The senator loved his view of the working home of Congress, arguably one of the most architecturally iconic structures in the nation.

He was musing about the morning's HELP Committee meeting and feeling pretty good about how it went. The FDA was a mess before Allisyn took over and completely overhauled the agency for the better. He was particularly pleased, since she was his recommendation to the president for the position of commissioner a little over two years ago.

Gradison had a background in health care law and met Allisyn when she gave a talk at a conference on medical research regulatory issues. The FDA problems were at a critical point at the time, and it was clear the then commissioner needed to be replaced. Gradison was so impressed with the depth of Allisyn's knowledge on the issue he immediately proposed her as a potential candidate. Who better to right the ship, he argued in support of her appointment, than someone with Allisyn's research background, regulatory expertise—and a Nobel Prize.

The president was equally impressed and Allisyn was interested in a change from research. A huge hit with the FDA staff, she sailed through the confirmation process. The rest, as they say, is history.

And her report today validated my recommendation, he thought.

Just then there was a knock on the partially open door. The senator looked up. It was Seth Krewe, his chief of staff.

Gradison and Krewe were long-time friends since they first met as college roommates. Although attending different law schools, they maintained a close friendship. Their professional lives diverged after graduation, but only temporarily. It was actually Krewe who got Gradison interested in politics, so it was natural that the senator tapped his long-time friend and colleague for the position as his chief of staff.

"Free to talk?"

"Sure. Come on in. I was just thinking about today's report. How do you feel it went?"

"Couldn't have been any better. Well, maybe not Lancaster's typical buffoonery, even though the good doctor handled it pretty easily."

"Yeah, but it did add a little spice to the proceedings."

Krewe took a seat. "Mm-hmm. I knew she was quick on her feet, but that was really impressive…in a funny sort of way. Besides, the old coot had it coming."

Gradison nodded. "Funny thing is, he probably didn't even realize it."

"Probably. Anyway, I think McLoren's report was spot on. From the little I've heard afterward, everyone's pretty happy with how she's turned the FDA around."

"Good thing, since I recommended her for the position. Not so much, I'm afraid, if things turned out otherwise."

"Speaking of which," said Krewe as he leaned forward in his chair, "I met with key members of the party last evening and they're convinced you're a lock as their presidential nominee next year."

"Really?" As a second term senator who served on a number of subcommittees, Gradison had occasionally thought about this possibility but was always reluctant to enter the fray.

"Come on, Senator. It's not like you and I have never discussed this. It seems now is the right time. You have high voter approval ratings and the growing support of the party. To top it all off, the other party's front runner has some issues making him vulnerable, not to mention his grating temperament and lack of any charisma."

"Hmm. You do make a compelling case. Still…"

"Seriously. With your experience in economics and health care law, this is a great opportunity to really make an impact. And given the ground level support developing, I think it's time for you to step out of the political shadows."

"Perhaps we differ there a bit, Seth. We both know you're much more comfortable than I am in the political arena."

Krewe shrugged but didn't disagree.

Gradison wasn't aware how true his statement really was. It was Krewe himself who had secretly cajoled party leaders into choosing Gradison over more politically experienced candidates in the first place, something Gradison himself had never considered pursuing.

"You owe it to the people of this country to take us in a new direction, Carlton."

Gradison nodded with a subtle, twisted smile. "You may be right, Seth. Perhaps it is time. But only if the support is there."

Krewe got up to leave. "Oh, it's definitely there all right. It's what I heard last night." He had a satisfied smile on his face.

"Then it seems I have something to really think about."

CHAPTER

FIVE

After the Senate hearing, Allisyn returned to her office to review emails and return phone calls. She had asked Ginger not to schedule any meetings for the afternoon. She anticipated being worn down by what she thought might be a taxing Q&A from the committee members. With the exception of the Mississippi senator's bombastic questioning, she had been pleasantly surprised how smoothly and non-confrontational the hearing went. Despite her relative euphoria, she was exhausted both physically and mentally. She decided to make it a shortened day and head on home.

Although her office was at the FDA's main campus in Silver Spring, Maryland, slightly north of the D.C. line, she had chosen to live in the District when she accepted the agency position. Having attended medical school at Georgetown University, she held a fondness for the nation's capital.

She quickly settled on a neighborhood in Southwest Washington. It was close to the D.C. waterfront and only a few blocks from Nationals Baseball Park. The area had undergone significant gentrification over the last several years. Like many of the buildings in the area, hers was converted from a dated housing project to a modernized, high-end condominium structure. The D.C. Metro was directly across the street and trendy new restaurants and bars seemed to be springing up on a regular basis.

Luckily, Allisyn's search was brief. One of the more recently renovated buildings had a vacancy on the fourth floor and she jumped on it. She converted the smaller of the two bedrooms into a study which doubled as a guest room, with a portable bed as needed. Her bedroom was larger, with a high-end bathroom design. An adequately sized kitchen with gourmet cooking appliances accompanied the dining area. The adjoining living room featured a large, floor to ceiling window which afforded an extraordinary view of the waterfront and the Arena Stage Performing Arts Center, a key selling point for Allisyn, along with the enclosed parking area.

To top it off, she was an easy walk from the National Mall and surrounding stores, restaurants, and entertainment venues, weather permitting.

When Allisyn arrived at her condo, she quickly showered and pulled on a pair of comfortable sweats. Even though it was a little early for dinner, she was pretty hungry. She had skipped lunch after the hearing, so she foraged for some leftovers in the fridge.

When finished, she grabbed a glass of wine and collapsed on her favorite chair. She sat sideways, legs draped over an armrest and facing the large window with the great view. New Orleans style jazz in the background, she was deep into a novel she had started a while back when her cell phone rang. She grabbed her phone, looked at the screen and smiled. It was her niece Megan, a medical resident at Georgetown University Hospital.

Allisyn and Megan shared a rapport not typical of their familial ties. When Allisyn's older sister and single mother Sarah tragically died of an accidental drug overdose at the age of twenty, their parents assumed responsibility for raising Megan. Since Allisyn was only four when Megan was born, the two children were so close in age they eventually developed a bond more akin to sisters than aunt and niece. Neither had any memory of Sarah, and as they became older and learned the truth, their friendship was strengthened by the emotional burden each carried in their own way.

"Hey there, girl!" said Allisyn. "How's my favorite resident doing?"

"Exhausted. I had in-house call last weekend and haven't gotten out of the hospital before ten every night this week. Good thing I'm off this weekend, though. Otherwise, they'd have to admit me as a patient."

"Very funny, Megs. Wait till next year. It'll be even worse. Same patient load or more, and you'll need to squeeze in prepping for the Boards."

"Great. Thanks a lot. I call my aunt for a healthy dose of sympathy and this is what I get?"

Allisyn laughed.

"Seriously, Alli. I thought maybe we could get together this weekend for lunch or dinner. I really miss our regular chats."

Although their relationship evolved as they matured, one thing remained from childhood. Megan was the only person Allisyn allowed to call her "Alli."

"You're on. What day works best?"

"I have to go in for Grand Rounds Saturday morning and they expect us to stay for the stale sandwiches and chips. Woohoo. I plan on crashing afterward."

"Sunday then. Lunch or dinner?"

Megan hesitated briefly. "Lunch okay?"

"Lunch it is. What're you up for? Italian, Chinese—"

"Actually, I'd love a nice juicy burger, fries and a cold beer. Maybe two."

"Sounds like a plan. How about the Tombs? Shouldn't be crowded on a Sunday. Say, noon?"

"Perfect. Unless I sleep right through till Monday in time for morning rounds."

"Mm-hmm. I don't think so. That's not like the Megs I know and love."

"Ha-ha! See ya then. Ciao."

"Ditto."

21

After the call, Allisyn finished the last of her wine and smiled to herself.

I hope we never stop bantering with each other like we did as teenagers.

———————

Allisyn parked her car along Prospect Street in Georgetown a block from the corner of 36th Street. The intersection of the two is the site of a steep set of iconic stone steps between two buildings leading down to M Street below. The staircase was built in 1895 and is now known as the "Exorcist Steps" made famous by its legendary role in the 1973 horror film, *The Exorcist.*

Immediately across the street from the top of the staircase is the 1789 Restaurant housed in a mid-nineteenth century, Federal-style townhouse named for the year Georgetown University was founded. What was especially important to Georgetown students, however—both past and present—was the building's basement. The Tombs was a rathskeller-style bar and eatery referencing the T.S. Eliot poem, *Bustopher Jones.* A favorite haunt of students, the winding brick staircase led down to the pub, with its elaborate polished wood bar and tables. The walls were covered with a plethora of photos and sketches of university life over the years. The mantle of a magnificent stone fireplace was encircled with rowing paddles inscribed with the names and dates of various crew competitions. Music played in the background, often tunes from the sixties and seventies. It was almost guaranteed you would hear the Beatles' *Hey Jude* at least once during your visit.

On any given Friday or Saturday night, the line to enter the establishment could be seen winding from the bottom of the steps all the way up to and often for a distance along the sidewalk above. On a Sunday afternoon, however, waiting was a rare occurrence.

Megan was standing on the sidewalk at the top of the steps when Allisyn approached. They hugged with genuine affection.

"So you didn't sleep through our date," teased Allisyn.

Her niece grinned. "Uh, almost."

"Let's go eat," Allisyn said, putting her arm around Megan's shoulder.

Sure enough, there was no wait to be seated when they went down the steps. They devoured their meals while sipping beer during a varied conversation.

"Where did you park?" asked Megan when they had finished and left the restaurant.

"Just around the corner. But I'd rather walk."

"To my place? You do know it's all the way on the other side of the campus and several blocks beyond, right?"

"No problem."

"Then I'll drive you back to your car."

"Uh-uh. I need the exercise. Besides, I'm not much older than you...remember?"

They laughed and set out walking casually.

"So I saw a replay of your Senate report," said Megan. "Fabulous. And your exchange with the senator? Priceless."

"Lancaster?"

"Yeah. One for the ages. How did you keep a straight face when you referenced Alexander Fleming and he said Sir Ian?"

Allisyn chuckled. "It wasn't easy."

"I bet." Megan paused. "Seriously, you've really done a phenomenal job getting the place straightened out. I mean, I don't know all the details but from what I've read, there were plenty of problems."

"Uh-huh. From a regulatory perspective, it was a disaster."

Megan didn't react right away. "So I've always meant to ask. How did you decide to give up research for the FDA in the first place? Don't know why, but you never talked with me about it."

"No reason. I mean no reason why I never went into detail with you about it." She paused and looked around. "This place is incredible. The campus has exploded with buildings."

"You changed the subject, Alli," said Megan in a mock scolding tone.

"Sorry. Well, after the Nobel ceremony, I was wondering how much more I could accomplish in research. And I kinda felt ready for a change, a new challenge. So much of what I did required knowledge of all the regulatory requirements for good research. I thought maybe I could contribute to fixing the FDA and help people by facilitating the approval of new treatment modalities."

As they walked, Allisyn intermittently pointed out what had existed prior to many of the new buildings which had more recently been constructed in their place.

As they approached the University Hospital, Allisyn stopped and pointed to the Yates Field House. It was built on the site of a running track featured in *The Exorcist* where a police detective played by Lee J. Cobb had a conversation with a university priest.

Allisyn laughed when Megan admitted to never having seen the movie.

After a brief silence, Megan reverted to their previous conversation about Allisyn and the FDA. "And now? Are you happy with how it's turned out? I mean how you feel about the change personally. Nobody can argue with how you've improved the FDA as a government agency."

Allisyn nodded slowly. "Yeah, for the most part." Her mind immediately flashed back to her conversation with Constance Vasquez before her Congressional report. "I just don't enjoy the politics."

Megan jerked her head back. "Politics? What does politics have to do with the FDA's role in approving medical devices and treatments?"

"Everything in Washington and its environs is affected by politics, Megs." Allisyn sighed. "It's just the way it is and what irks me about the job."

"Hmm…I guess I can understand why it would be annoying."

"What about you? Are you thinking of specializing after your residency?"

"As a matter of fact, I'm leaning towards an Infectious Disease Fellowship with research, like you've done. Maybe get involved in the CDC. What do you think?"

Allisyn hesitated. She was keenly aware of the influence her status as a role model might have on Megan and wanted to be measured in her response. "Sounds interesting enough. My only advice is if you want research, don't rule out academics or even Pharma first. It's where you earn credibility. You can always get to government work later, whether it's the CDC or some other branch...If you still want it."

Megan nodded. "Makes sense. Anyway, right now I'm concentrating on getting a fellowship. I figure the rest will come later."

"Smart. Just be sure any program you consider has a strong research component. It's a definite must have."

"Right." She hesitated. "Uh, you won't mind if I run my options by you, eh?"

"Of course not. I'd be a little disappointed if you didn't."

They had just about reached the other side of the campus. The house Megan shared with three other residents was still several blocks beyond Reservoir Road.

"I think I'll stop here," said Allisyn, "and work my way back."

"Thanks so much, Alli, for lunch... and the advice. We have to find time to do this more often."

"You bet." Allisyn reached out and they warmly hugged before she headed back to her car.

She ambled back across the campus and continued to marvel at the expansion and landscape change occurring over the years. Reflecting on her conversation with Megan, she realized she hadn't been completely honest with her niece about leaving research for the FDA. In fact, she never admitted to anyone the

25

role her former fiancé played in her decision to leave her research position in California and move across the country to get away. Then again, no one—not even Megan—knew how much of an emotional toll her failed relationship had taken.

CHAPTER

SIX

Allisyn sat in her office at the end of a long day, reviewing the stack of phone messages her assistant Ginger had left for her before leaving. She was still seething from her disturbing conversation with Vasquez and was flipping through the messages to distract herself. As was her usual custom, she prioritized them before starting the tedious process of returning the calls. This often lasted into the early evening. Halfway through the stack, she stopped and stared disbelievingly at the name in front of her. It was accompanied by a note to return the call as soon as possible.

They hadn't really spoken since she left Rome. Sure, they would occasionally see each other at scientific conferences, but she always avoided any meaningful interaction between them, struggling but always successful at overcoming her emotions.

This time was different. Perhaps because it was a direct request to speak with her rather than a chance meeting. She closed her eyes and tried to think of a reason not to call back.

It was after eight when Allisyn finished her phone calls. All but one. She had put Paul Westin's message at the end of the priority list but knew returning his call was unavoidable. They hadn't been in contact since she became FDA Commissioner, save for his congratulatory email which she answered with a simple "Thanks."

She dialed the number, consciously hoping there would be no answer, postponing the conversation at least until tomorrow.

Unfortunately, he answered after only two rings. "Hello?"

Allisyn froze. She couldn't speak. Everything she had tried to forget now came crashing back around her at the sound of his voice. The challenge of inquiry and investigation, the thrill of discovery, the excitement of reward, and the romanticism of the Eternal City. And, yes, even the guilt and shame of betrayal.

"Paul?" She didn't identify herself, but he immediately recognized her voice. She knew he would.

"How are you, Allisyn? Pretty well, it seems. Apparently, you've really taken to your new position. I watched your report to Congress, and I must say the results you've achieved since joining the FDA are impressive."

"Thanks. I see you've been keeping busy yourself at Nu-Genomix." Allisyn felt uneasy at how awkwardly formal this conversation seemed. She wondered if he felt the same, but it quickly became clear he didn't.

"I was wondering," he said, "if you and I could meet privately for lunch or dinner."

She hesitated briefly. "I don't think that would be a good idea, Paul. I don't want to go there."

"No, no. I'm sorry. It's not personal, not about us. I'm not looking to rekindle anything, Allisyn. So much has happened since our joint research ended that I thought it might be a nice idea if we could catch up professionally with each other. Besides, I have a proposition to discuss with you."

She bristled at the thought. "What kind of proposition?"

"I'll be speaking at a conference on genomics at Georgetown University and I thought you might be interested in joining me for a panel discussion. I think it would make for an interesting forum. After all, it's your medical school alma mater and Washington is your home now."

She didn't respond.

"So? What do you think?" he asked, breaking the silence.

"I don't know. It might be a little awkward for both of us."

"Really? I thought we agreed we could still have civil professional interactions. Providing the perspectives of private industry and government regulation on genomic research should make for some provocative questions from the audience. What do you say?"

She was accustomed to receiving speaking engagement requests on a regular basis, but a one on one with Westin caused her to hesitate. "I guess I could participate."

"Great. I'll have my assistant get in touch with yours first thing in the morning about the date and time. Now, about dinner—"

"I'll pass," she said abruptly. "Let's keep this formal and stick with the conference only, please. No offense. Okay?"

"Sure. None taken." He hesitated. "I do have one other issue I'd prefer to discuss in person, although I doubt we'll get the opportunity at the conference."

"We can do it now. What's the issue?"

"The Nu-Genomix application for our gene therapy treatment for heart failure. You are familiar with it, yes?"

How disingenuous of him to even suggest the possibility I might not know about it. I even referenced it at the Senate hearing.

"Of course I am."

"Then I'd like to discuss the Advisory Committee's recommendation."

She sighed. "I've already reviewed the report and I'm fully aware of their positive view of your work. What specifically do you want to discuss?"

"Then you know the committee recommended our therapy be considered for an expedited priority review. I was wondering if the CBER review team is moving forward with their recommendation. After all, our product does employ a novel technology which is safe and more effective than current treatments. The committee even designated it a potential breakthrough therapy."

Allisyn frowned. "You should make such a request directly to Dr. Francke, leader of the review team."

"Of course. As we plan to do. I was only hoping you could look into it yourself and ensure they're moving the review along expeditiously as recommended by your own Advisory Committee."

Her back stiffened. "I have full confidence in the team's ability to move on your application as appropriate. Including expediting the review if they feel it's warranted. The team doesn't need me to remind them."

"Of course, of course," said Westin. "I just thought—"

"Sorry. It's not a good idea for me to interfere with the review given our respective positions and our past work history together. It's important for me to maintain an appropriate distance to avoid any inference of conflict of interest. In fact, I don't believe this conversation should even be taking place."

"Really now, Allisyn. Our paths have been divergent long enough. A simple professional discussion about the science surrounding our research couldn't possibly be mistaken for collusion."

"Collusion? Who said anything about collusion? That's not what I'm talking about. Given our…professional history, suspicion of data bias and conflict of interest is not the least bit far-fetched. It behooves both of us to avoid such a perception."

"I honestly think you're overstating the potential concerns about impropriety. After all, you are the commissioner. I don't think anybody would consider it improper for you to take an interest in products under review."

Allisyn rubbed her forehead between thumb and finger. *I can't believe this conversation is really happening.*

"I'm certain you're aware of the policy stipulating the commissioner is recused from the actual decision making of the evaluation process. Such specific activity is the sole purview of the staff experts reviewing the application."

"Of course I'm aware of it, Allisyn. I'm only asking for the commissioner's endorsement of her own Advisory Committee's positive evaluation and recommendation to expedite the process."

She could feel the warmth rising up her neck into her face and a dryness in her throat. Her irritation had turned to indignation. For him to make this request was well outside the boundaries of propriety. Especially in view of the agency's past problems with industry bias and their past work history together.

"That's simply not going to happen, Paul. And now it's best this discussion ends right here. Goodbye."

"But—"

"No. This conversation is over." And she hung up without waiting for a further response.

Allisyn was a bundle of mixed emotions. She angrily pushed her chair back from the desk, almost hitting the credenza behind her, and stood to leave. *Dammit! I never should have agreed to the conference invitation in the first place.*

CHAPTER

SEVEN

At six foot-three, trim and upright in stature, Julian Shawe was a commanding presence. A full head of dark gray hair with subtle streaks of silver and a strong baritone voice with a hint of a British accent added to his imperious aura.

After attending business school, Shawe turned an inheritance from his father into an entrepreneur's dream. He acquired a small data management company from a pair of struggling IT graduates and aggressively turned it into one of the most successful biotech firms around. Although he initially used the company to generate huge profits through the production of GMOs—Genetically Modified Organisms—for the purpose of food production, the company was now fully dedicated to the research and development of human gene therapy. As president, CEO and board chairman of Nu-Genomix, Shawe left no doubt who was in charge.

The Nu-Genomix research facility was located in Research Triangle Park. RTP, as it is often called, is one of the largest such concentrations of diverse research firms in the world and is wedged between the North Carolina cities of Durham, Raleigh and Chapel Hill. The company was RTP's most recent and fastest growing biotech addition.

Shawe was getting anxious, and he had called an impromptu meeting with Dr. Paul Westin to determine if additional action was needed to get their gene therapy approved by the FDA.

Westin was director of research for the biotech firm and principal investigator for their heart failure gene therapy investigational study and clinical trial program.

Joining them was Jason Tinley, Shawe's "special assistant," as he referred to him. Tinley didn't have a place on the Nu-Genomix organizational chart. He didn't even have a formal job description. And his name wasn't found in any company document. What Tinley did have was a particularly keen ability to get things done—on Shawe's behalf—which were not identified in any strategic plan, annual report or corporate tactical action item list. Whenever Shawe spoke of him, he would simply reference a "special assignment." Everyone knew not to ask what it might be.

Tinley had the stereotypical appearance of a special ops warrior. Straight-faced and squared-jawed, he rarely showed any emotion. He was more than six feet tall, broad-shouldered, and trim but visibly muscular. He had a military style crew cut and consistently kept his shirt collar turned up.

The "special assistant" had a pretty sordid background. He had been in the military but left when his tour of duty was up, bitter because his bid to enter special ops training was denied. Apparently, his psychological profile was questionable—for want of another way of describing it. After discharge, he served in a number of mercenary roles in several politically unstable African countries. He quickly learned to do whatever it took to achieve an objective and get the job done. And equally important, to cover his tracks and watch his back.

Shawe met him while attending a conference in Malaysia on emerging biotech companies in Southeast Asia, where Tinley had been assigned as a security agent. Shawe struck up several conversations with Tinley, finding him a particularly unsavory character. Oddly enough, however, they got along better than expected, and he started thinking the kind of skills Tinley possessed, as offensive as they might be, could come in handy in certain situations. He felt his own business bravado melded perfectly with Tinley's ability to disregard any sense of displeasure for a task needing to be done, no matter how distasteful. Shawe offered him a very attractive salary, and since then, Tinley had proven to be incredibly resourceful and highly valuable. Shawe considered him one of his best hires. He always delivered and never disappointed.

Shawe's usual venue for a meeting with his inner circle was his office, a spacious room generously decorated with priceless artifacts from around the world and furnished with exquisitely crafted teakwood and leather furniture. Several floor to ceiling built-in bookcases held numerous tomes covering diverse topics. This was all accentuated by a 180-degree glass enclosure providing a spectacular view of the meticulously maintained landscaping outside.

As he often did when the weather cooperated, however, Shawe chose to have their discussion outside in his personal garden. Typically, he would dabble around the flowers and plants, sprucing and trimming with a pair of shears as they talked. It might appear as though he was disinterested in the conversation, but he never missed a word.

"I'd like to see where we stand with our application, gentlemen," said Shawe.

Westin spoke up. "The CBER review team—"

"Say again?" said Tinley. "What does CBER mean? I forgot."

"The Center for Biologics Evaluation and Review. Their team reviews every FDA application, all the data, and makes a recommendation for approval or requests further studies to substantiate a request for approval."

"Oh. Right."

Westin did a slight eye roll. "So their review team has received our responses to their initial questions regarding our research methodology, but we have no feedback from them as of yet. However, when I spoke to the team leader, Dr. Francke, yesterday, she indicated there likely would be some additional questions they would be submitting regarding our data before we meet a second time."

Shawe kept stopping here and there to prune a plant as they meandered through the garden. "Any problems?" he asked without looking up.

"Not really. This is pretty standard follow-up to the initial application meeting. Of course, we'll have to see how they react to the responses we provide them."

Shawe continued his landscaping. "What's the timeline on this?"

"Hard to say. They usually don't provide any expectations for how quickly they move on these submissions. They do work as expeditiously as possible, however, given the volume of ongoing applications they're dealing with. And the complex nature of our treatment and the data required to support it also needs to be considered. On the positive side, it's to our benefit their Advisory Committee has recommended expedited review as a breakthrough treatment, which should make the review much faster than the standard evaluation. We'll know more when they give us feedback on our answers to their questions. Once the NDA—New Drug Application—is approved, we can begin production and market the product as a viable therapy. Then we can start the testing on conditions other than heart failure." He paused. "Nevertheless, I do have some concerns."

Shawe abruptly turned his head and glanced up. "Concerns? Like what?"

"According to our intel, we've been way ahead of any competitor from the beginning. And unless something negative delays the CBER review, we have enough of a head start to negate any serious challenge. If we do get delayed much further, however, it may pose more of a problem. The sooner we get FDA approval, the better."

Shawe stopped his gardening and stood up straight to face them. "Hmm. It seems imperative, then, that we leverage the lead we already have so we can move forward with production.

We certainly can't allow anyone else to surpass us in getting our product to market. Otherwise, the negative effect on our financial projections would be...let's just say, not pretty. And our investors will not be happy." He paused, stroking his chin. "Were you able to meet with Dr. McLoren regarding her cooperation in achieving expedited review and approval?"

Westin sighed. "I broached the topic with her recently when I invited her to join me to speak on a panel at an upcoming conference. Unfortunately, the discussion didn't go well."

He described his entire conversation with Allisyn, including her adversarial posture to her getting involved in the process. "She insinuated her endorsement of the therapy would be akin to collusion with us and indicative of both industry and agency bias."

"Any reasonable chance you could persuade her otherwise with further discussion?"

"I actually tried to convince her she was overstating her concern, but she became pretty indignant. And she ended the conversation. I'm fairly certain she's not going to budge from her position...at least without some additional incentive."

They came to a little patio area with white metal garden benches and Shawe sat. Westin and Tinley followed suit.

Shawe hesitated, gazing up and pursing his lips briefly. "Then it seems time to proceed with the contingency plans we've made in case this process seemed to be stalling out." He turned toward Tinley. "Jason, where do we stand with the assignment we discussed?"

"I recently acquired the necessary information to make our proposal indeed compelling."

"Good. Tell us a little about the senator's chief of staff."

Tinley pulled a small notebook from his jacket pocket. He routinely used it to record notes on the intel he gathered. "Krewe and Gradison met as college roommates and became really tight with each other. In fact, Gradison met his future wife at the same time, and all three have remained pretty close since then. Gradison and Krewe went to different law schools after graduation and in different professional directions. Gradison returned to his home state to practice law, specializing in health care law and regulations. Krewe stayed in D.C. At first, he worked in the legal department for a large lobbying firm. But then he left to form his own independent lobbying practice. Apparently. he was pretty good at it, too, from what I could gather. He became sort of a legend in the Washington lobbying world, building one of the most successful practices in record time."

"A little unusual, isn't it?" said Westin.

Tinley tilted his head. "How so?"

"I mean, most successful lobbyists usually come from the ranks of congressional staffers, leveraging their legislative relationships. Not having served in government, Krewe didn't have those connections."

"Hmm," said Shawe. "Even more impressive that he achieved what he did in such an unorthodox way."

Westin frowned. "He left a highly lucrative lobbying practice to enter government service as Gradison's chief of staff? Odd, don't you think?"

Tinley shrugged. "Anyway, as the story goes, it was actually Krewe who encouraged his friend to enter politics and at the same time convinced the party leadership to appoint his pal to a vacated Senate seat. He later went on to successfully engineer Gradison's subsequent election to the position. The new senator returned the favor when he insisted his friend serve as his chief of staff, and Krewe has been there ever since. Conventional wisdom has it he holds a pretty strong sway over the senator. And if you can believe all the rumors going around, it's Krewe himself who's behind Gradison's run for president."

"Now it all makes sense," said Westin. "Sounds like Krewe's exchanged his cash flow for a power grab."

Tinley nodded. "Probably had already made a fortune from his lobbying days anyway."

"So what's your play on this guy?" said Shawe. He reached down to pull a few stray weeds from around some flowers.

"As I delved into Krewe's background, I came across a young politician by the name of Maxwell whom Krewe befriended in Washington. This guy was in law school at the time and met Krewe at a seminar. They hit it off and Krewe became a mentor of sorts."

"Where does he come in?"

"It seems Krewe would become quite talkative after a couple of drinks, and discretion apparently went out the window when they socialized. Turns out Krewe was involved in several border-line illegal campaign contribution deals which he was able to sweep under the rug. Only problem was he shared all of it with this guy Maxwell. And I obtained some juicy details about Krewe's misadventures from him."

"And this . . . source was willing to share all this with you for no specific reason?" asked Shawe. "So easily?"

"Mm-hmm. Once I threatened to expose what I knew about the cocaine parties he and his friends regularly engage in."

"Ahh, I see. Interesting approach, Jason." Shawe stopped his gardening and stood. "Let us know how your meeting with Krewe goes. If your conversation with the senator's chief of staff is productive and has the desired outcome, our investors will be quite pleased indeed."

As the three parted ways, Shawe was thinking about his "special assistant.'" *Always delivers and never disappoints.*

CHAPTER

EIGHT

Seth Krewe walked to his car parked on a quiet street several blocks from his house.

He was about to start the car when the passenger door opened and a stranger quickly slipped into the seat and pulled the door closed. He sported a crew cut and turned up collar.

"Huh!" gasped Krewe. "What the fuck? Get the hell out of my car!" He reached for his cell phone.

"Please, Mr. Krewe," said Jason Tinley. "I'm not here to harm you, I only—"

"How do you know my name?"

Tinley ignored Krewe's question. "As I was going to say, I would just like to make a proposal."

"Proposal? Who are you?"

"I represent a number of business associates."

"Business associates? This is ridiculous. I'm calling the police."

"I wouldn't advise it, Seth." Tinley conspicuously pulled back one side of his jacket, exposing the butt end of a pistol tucked into his pants waistband.

Krewe's eyes grew wide and he dropped the phone on the floorboard.

"Now, as I was saying, I represent a number of business associates who share a common interest in the future of health care in this country and want to support individuals who are in a position to help improve care for our citizens."

"W-w-what does it have to do with me?" Krewe's hands were trembling and his breathing quickened. Small beads of sweat were forming on his forehead.

"Yes, yes. About my proposal." Tinley let his jacket fall back, covering the gun. "It turns out my associates are enamored with Senator Gradison as a presidential candidate, given his extensive background in health care law and progressive views on the future of health care. In fact, his recommendation of Dr. McLoren for FDA commissioner, who has reformed the agency in exemplary fashion, is an example of the kind of forward-looking approach we need."

Krewe slumped in his seat, his face taking on an ashen hue.

Tinley paused briefly. "Now then, as I was saying…oh yes, about the senator's progressive views on health care. This has never been more important than in today's scientific environment, which is rapidly generating innovative and exciting forms of medical treatment which can provide new hope for many unfortunate individuals."

Krewe's color appeared to be returning slightly, and his breathing slowed down.

"You're looking a little better, Seth, I'm glad to see. Now, about my proposal. Nu-Genomix is a company which has developed just such an innovative treatment under review for approval by the FDA. And my associates have provided substantial financial support for its development. However, as with such developments, competitors are always lurking around the corner, so time is of the essence in ensuring the Nu-Genomix treatment is approved so patients who have failed traditional treatments can be helped . . . and my associates' investments are protected."

Krewe's gaze was diverted away from the intruder.

"Are you still with me, Seth?"

Krewe's only response was to look back over at him.

"Good, then. My associates are prepared to provide substantial campaign finance support for the senator if Dr. McLoren could be . . . let's say, encouraged to assist in expediting the approval process for the Nu-Genomix application so it can be made available to needy patients in a timely fashion."

Krewe frowned, slowly shaking his head and murmuring. "The senator . . . would never even consider—"

"Let me clarify, Seth. We certainly don't expect the senator himself to speak with Dr. McLoren. You, on the other hand, as his trusted adviser and confidante, can intervene with the commissioner on his behalf. Given your lobbying expertise, I'm sure you would be quite persuasive in getting her to understand how her assistance could reinforce the senator's—uh, future president's—confidence in her continuing as the FDA commissioner."

Tinley paused and leaned slightly toward Krewe, staring directly into his eyes.

"Speaking of lobbying, Mr. Krewe, in case you don't find my proposal quite incentive enough to cooperate, I'm sure you wouldn't appreciate a public disclosure of certain, uh, let's say questionable, campaign financing deals engineered by you which were borderline at best, if not actually illegal and deftly covered up. Some of which were actually to benefit the senator's own campaign. I think you would agree his bid for president would sustain a devastating, perhaps fatal blow, if this information somehow surfaced. Politically speaking, of course. And I don't think the senator would take kindly to having his political aspirations, and yours as well, go up in flames over such a scandal involving his chief of staff and long-time personal friend."

Slumping against the car door, Krewe was silent.

Tinley paused for maximum effect before continuing. "Now here's some good news, Mr. Krewe. None of this will matter, because it will never come to light as long as you accomplish one simple task. Convince Commissioner McLoren to ensure approval of the Nu-Genomix application for its gene therapy product, and soon. Accomplish this one task, game over, and we all win. Put another way, you help us by helping to get the Nu-

Genomix application approved, and we help you by, as the saying goes, letting sleeping dogs lie. And the senator gets financial campaign support as an added benefit."

Tinley stopped and waited for a response.

Krewe didn't move immediately. He slowly turned his head away from the car door window it was leaning against. Without saying a word, he looked at Tinley through drooping eyelids, his shoulders slumped and lips slightly parted with the sound of slow, heavy breathing.

"I'm going to assume you're in full agreement with our proposal, then," resumed Tinley. "And one more thing. I urge you to keep our little, uh, conversation today just between the two of us." He pulled his jacket back, again exposing the gun handle. "Otherwise, the consequences could be quite unpleasant. Now then, we'll expect some good news from the commissioner very soon, or the situation is guaranteed to quickly get ugly for you and the senator."

His task complete, Tinley exited the car, leaving Krewe speechless and alone.

CHAPTER

NINE

What does she want this time?

Allisyn arrived with time to spare for the early morning meeting requested by Constance Vasquez at the last minute the day before. She had no idea why the secretary wanted to meet again this soon after the Senate hearing with so little advance notification. And after their last meeting, she really wasn't looking forward to this one.

"You're probably wondering why I wanted to get together again this quickly," said the HHS secretary.

Allisyn simply nodded.

"Let me explain. After your well-received report to the HELP Committee, I decided to do some catching up on the more interesting new product applications the agency is working on and thought we might discuss a few."

Allisyn was skeptical but played along. "Any in particular?"

"The new immunotherapy for lung cancer seems to be a real breakthrough. Is it close to being approved?"

"Yes, I believe it is. Their study results are indeed impressive. Should have the CBER report shortly."

"Wonderful. And I've heard the new insulin pump is a real improvement over current technology."

"Uh-huh. It's fast tracked for approval. I think it'll make a real difference for patients."

Vasquez hesitated. "What about this new form of gene therapy? You know, the one from the company you referred to during your report to the HELP Committee. I forget the name."

"Nu-Genomix?"

"Right. You would think I'd remember such a catchy name. How's their application going?"

"If you mean Gen-X, their pre-marketing designation for the gene therapy for heart failure with a genetic cause, it's still in evaluation. I suspect they'll come up with a sexier marketing name if it's approved. So far, our team is looking at it favorably. They still need to clarify some additional data before making a final determination."

"I suppose you're pretty familiar with it yourself. I mean it was your field of research, right?"

"Related, yes. But this is something new—creating a synthetic gene. Different from my work. It hadn't been previously tested, this being its first completed clinical trial."

Vasquez leaned back in her chair, folding her arms. "It's generated quite a buzz around here. It seems several members of Congress have a particular interest in the therapy. Apparently, they're better informed than me on the science surrounding it."

Allisyn's eyes narrowed. "What kind of buzz?"

"From what I hear, they're questioning what the delay is in approving it."

Now Allisyn tensed in her chair and tightly gripped the arm rests. "Delay? There's no delay. The review is being carried out as per protocol. I'm sure you can appreciate their therapy is a complex treatment. It's important the supporting data is fully vetted and validated, which takes time. I wouldn't call that a delay."

"You don't have to get all defensive, Allisyn. I'm not implying by any means there's been an intentional delay. I only heard the agency's own Technical Advisory Committee has already recommended expedited review, presumably leading to approval. I was simply curious as to when the review and approval would happen."

"Correct, but it doesn't lessen the degree of detailed evaluation required by the CBER review team. Besides, such a preliminary recommendation doesn't guarantee approval. The final determination is made by CBER. You certainly wouldn't want anything less than the thorough scrutiny which follows our protocol."

"Of course. I understand, and I'm not suggesting otherwise. To the layperson, however, expedited means moving along faster than normal. I guess some of the interested parties are wondering—"

"Wondering? About what?"

The secretary's neck stiffened and she scowled at being interrupted. "If you must know, Allisyn, I've received some inquiries as to why you can't help the review process move along more quickly, since this is your area of research expertise. . . . I was actually wondering the same thing myself. After all, you are an expert in all this, and it seems to be a valid question."

Allisyn frowned and shook her head slightly. "I see. So what are you suggesting?"

"Perhaps you could look into how the review is going, maybe push it along a little. I would think that should be within your purview, would it not?"

"You do know it's policy for the commissioner to keep any specific review process at arm's length, right?

"Of course. And I know you're committed to maintaining the integrity of the entire process you've worked so hard to improve. However, I must admit there seems to be a reasonable justification for you to loosen up the restriction a bit given your expertise in this field. After all, it's likely you have as much or more knowledge about all this than anybody on your staff."

Allisyn felt her face warming and a tightness in her throat. "The review process is standardized, Constance, and the members of all the CBER review committees are well-versed in application review and data analysis. They have my full confidence."

"Please, I'm not implying otherwise. I simply think it would seem reasonable for you to get a little more involved than you otherwise would."

Vasquez leaned forward, closer to Allisyn, and put both hands flat on her desk, Her tone of voice was now firmer. "Not just reasonable. I strongly advise you to intervene and expedite the review and approval. It would be the prudent course of action for you to take."

Allisyn was stunned and speechless at what she'd just heard. She couldn't believe what was being asked of her, nor did she have any clue why. What she did know was acquiescing would go against her own protocol. Even though she had no intention of complying, she knew there was no point in debating this further with her boss until she could figure it out.

"I'll think about it."

Vasquez leaned back again and crossed her arms once more. "When you do, be sure to consider all the ramifications of your decision. We don't want to breathe new life into previous allegations of overregulation. Concerns about delays in the availability to patients of important new treatments is certainly not a road we want to go down again. Once you give it more thought, I'm sure you'll realize it would be in your best interest, personally and career-wise, to do whatever you can to be considered proactive in supporting such new medical innovations. Especially this one. After all, we don't need an FDA commissioner who's not willing to visualize the future and make it a reality."

Angry and afraid of what she might say, Allisyn didn't dare respond. She was appalled by what she knew was inappropriate pressure to insert herself into the review process in such a manner. Even worse, she was offended by the veiled threat. After exchanging mutually perfunctory goodbyes with the secretary, Allisyn left without further discussion. By the time she returned to her office, she was still confused and upset about how the meeting had ended. It was clear what Vasquez was suggesting, but not so much why.

I wonder if she has some political motive.

CHAPTER

TEN

The conference was to be held in Gaston Hall, a 740-seat auditorium located within the Healy Building, the spired flagship structure of Georgetown University's main campus, located on a bluff overlooking the Potomac River. The ornately adorned interior of the venerable hall, with its balcony and decorated wood ceiling, had been the venue for innumerable events, having hosted a range of lecturers, guest speakers and dignitaries over the years.

Allisyn's cab pulled into Healy Circle, a circular drive immediately inside the university's main gate and fronting the building's main entrance. Prominently displayed in the center of the circle was a statue of the seated John Carroll, bishop and founder of the university in 1789. Although the medical school and hospital where Allisyn had been a student were located on the opposite side of the campus, she was perfectly familiar with this location. It served as a meeting place for all students, and its main gate opened to the Washington enclave which was Georgetown.

A shiver rippled through Allisyn as she climbed the Healy stone steps and entered the large entry foyer with its majestic wooden staircase leading to Gaston Hall. Her thoughts reverted fondly to days gone by.

She was immediately greeted by a university representative who she assumed recognized her from her photo in the conference brochure and escorted to the back stage area of the hall. There she was introduced to additional university representatives and dignitaries.

Paul Westin had already arrived, and they exchanged polite but curt greetings while they waited for the conference to begin. When advised by staff, they took their places in chairs centered on the stage. Each chair was angled between facing one another and the audience, with a podium off to one side. It was obvious from surveying the audience it was a packed house.

At the appointed time, Dean of the Medical School and Chair of the Department of Genetics Dr. Helena Greensworth welcomed all attendees and thanked both guests for their participation. She proceeded to provide a summary bio of each and offered several comments about their credentials. She stressed the work they had done together in genomic research, for which they had shared the Nobel Prize. They would each speak briefly on their respective topic, Westin on private, non-academic research, and Allisyn on the regulatory aspects. Their presentations would be followed by questions.

Westin spoke first and focused on the broad topic of the current state of genomic research. He mentioned only briefly the seminal research he and Allisyn had done together in the past. Although he referenced the research with which he had been more recently engaged at Nu-Genomics, he provided no specifics.

Allisyn spoke on the FDA's regulatory role in evaluating gene therapies being submitted for review. She emphasized the importance of balancing timely review with due diligence to ensure the scientific data supported approval and safety concerns were adequately addressed.

When they both finished, Dr. Greensworth opened the session up to questions from the audience. Most were follow-up queries on their specific talks. The two speakers were also asked for their opinions on which types of genetic disorders would be best suited for this mode of therapy, their pitfalls and potential successes.

Nearing the end of the allotted time, a young gentleman identifying himself as a resident at the university's hospital was recognized to pose a question. "Dr. Westin, could you address the potential for using this type of gene manipulation for non-disease purposes? So-called designer genes?"

Westin remained seated. "I believe you're referring to the concept of human genetic engineering, the elective introduction of engineered genes into an individual to produce specific desirable traits. In other words, not to make someone well from a particular disease process, but better than well by optimizing an attribute or capability. An example would be raising an individual from standard to peak levels of performance, say, in athletics or musical ability. Although our current focus is on using gene therapy to treat diseases when appropriate, there certainly is every reason to believe this technology could also be adapted to such elective enhancement at some point in the not too distant future."

Dr. Greensworth turned to Allisyn. "Dr. McLoren?"

Allisyn hesitated. She was somewhat taken aback and troubled by Westin's nonchalant approach to what they both knew was a complex and controversial issue. Concern among the scientific community and bioethicists over both the safety and social implications of such procedures was well known.

She stood up at the podium. "Let me first say there are no proposals currently before the FDA for consideration of such genetic manipulation or engineering for the purpose of non-disease enhancement. Nor are there any active studies currently under way for such purpose. At least to my knowledge. Regarding the feasibility of such an elective procedure, there are multiple concerns to address, making this a complex issue. Certainly, ongoing research has allowed the growth of genetic testing for non-pathologic traits and behaviors. Such as eye color, height, handedness and so forth. However, many traits which might be considered desirable to enhance are not the result of a single gene, but rather a complex interaction of multiple genes. Environmental, behavioral and nutritional factors often play a role as well. To say one can successfully predict the expression of a specific trait by introducing a mutated gene controlling the trait is at best a gross oversimplification. Until it is sorted out, if it ever is, extreme caution should be exercised in viewing this technology as a simple, routine way of changing a given individual's traits."

"With all due respect to Dr. McLoren," said Westin abruptly, without being asked to respond, "there is no reason combining such gene manipulation with modification of those other influential factors should not be available to those individuals who electively desire trait enhancement. Nor should we withhold it from them for artificial or unproven reasons once we have tested the technique. The fact is people currently undergo all manner of enhancement procedures. These include cosmetic surgery such as facelifts, hair implants, breast implants, risky weight loss surgery and others. Genetic enhancement is not much different. Dismissing the potential of this form of intervention simply because of complexity is contrary to the spirit of innovation and simply not forward-looking."

A few murmurs were audible among the audience and Dr. Greensworth quickly jumped in. "I think we can all agree this has been an interesting discussion, and I want to thank both—"

"Excuse me, but I feel I must respond to Dr. Westin's observations." Allisyn was flabbergasted and affronted by his last comment, both in content and tone. And she certainly didn't intend her terse proclamation to dispel such a perception on the part of those present. "I believe Dr. Westin is understating the complexity of this issue. There are factors at play beyond the technical capability and feasibility of elective genetic enhancement, not the least of which are ethical, legal and social considerations. Are we changing what is considered normal by enhancing or augmenting traits or functions meeting the definition of normal by current standards? And if genetic enhancement is elective, will it be available to all or only to those who can afford the expense? This goes to the question of undermining the principle of social equality. And although evaluation of the technical aspects of such an intervention falls under the purview of the FDA, genetic manipulation is likely to be unapproved for elective enhancement for the reasons stated. Which means they may be used off-label, bypassing effective FDA regulatory control." She paused. "And then there is the legal issue which arises when parents seek this type of enhancement for their children, negating their right for self-determination. Besides the risks and potential benefits of elective genetic manipulation, these ethical, moral and even legal issues must be thoroughly discussed before we consider its use for such purposes."

She stopped speaking, and the audience was hushed.

Dr. Greensworth took advantage of the pause to again attempt closure of the now contentious discourse. "This brings our conference to an end. I want to thank Doctors Westin and McLoren for taking the time to be with us today and provide some thought-provoking discussion."

Allisyn and Westin barely acknowledged each other before leaving separately.

Allisyn made her way quickly through the exiting throng. She ignored the numerous comments being exchanged among the conference attendees about the closing exchange they had just witnessed. Reaching the bottom of the steps of Gaston Hall, she heard a familiar voice from behind her.

"Alli, wait. Alli!"

Allisyn abruptly stopped and turned, eyes scanning the group. She smiled when she saw a hand waving and stepped off to the side.

Megan approached Allisyn with arms outstretched. She gave her quasi sister a quick hug, then pulled back. "You were awesome!"

Allisyn smiled weakly. "Thanks, Megs."

"What's with that asshole, anyway? Could he be any more arrogant and self-righteous?"

Allisyn shook her head, shrugging off her question. "I'm glad you could make it. Didn't you say you were on call?"

"Yeah, but I was able to make a last-minute shift swap with someone who owed me one. No way I was going to miss this if I could help it."

"Well, I appreciate the support."

"Seriously, Alli. You'd think Westin would be a little more deferential to you given you worked so closely together."

Overlooking her comment again, Allisyn turned her head. She gazed away for a few seconds, then turned back. "You got a few minutes?"

"Uh-huh. What's up?"

"Can you take a little walk?"

"Sure."

"Ever been to the Dahlgren Quadrangle?"

"No, never. I'm really not familiar with this side of the campus, sorry to say."

Allisyn led the way down a side road to the rear of the Healy Building, then left along a short walkway into a small, tree-lined brick plaza.

The Dahlgren Quadrangle marked the historic center of the Georgetown campus. It was enclosed on both sides by two of the oldest university buildings, with the back of the Healy Building at one end and the Dahlgren Chapel at the other end.

They sat together on a stone bench facing the chapel.

Allisyn stared at the small brick building of worship as she spoke. "When I was in med school, I often came here whenever I needed to clear my mind. Meditate, I guess you could say, although not in the formal sense. Or just to get away from it all. I found it especially helpful when things weren't going well, like when we lost a patient." She paused and nodded gently. "I always struggled with bad outcomes, you know? I often think it's why I moved on to research, to avoid getting emotionally involved with patients. I guess I rationalized it was still helping others through research without the personal involvement. I don't know."

Allisyn hesitated and lowered her gaze toward her hands folded in her lap. "I wasn't completely honest with you, Megs. About why I left my research position in California to take the FDA job. I mean, I didn't actually lie. I just didn't tell you the whole story. It's still . . . painful emotionally."

Megan glanced at Allisyn with concern and gently placed a hand on her arm. "It's okay, Alli. Whatever it is, it's okay."

Eyes misting, Allisyn looked up at her. "Before I left for my research stint at the University of Rome, Jordan and I had been discussing engagement. We knew the interim period would be a challenge for our relationship given the distance of separation, so we each committed to occasional trips back and forth to see each other. We went ahead and formalized our engagement, figuring we would make our wedding plans when I permanently returned after my two-year research project."

Allisyn felt a tightness in her throat and swallowed hard. "When Paul Westin and I were first working together at the University in Rome, we were strictly research collaborators, consumed by our work on a daily basis. When our efforts began to show promising results, the excitement level rose. The exhilaration of our work led to a more . . . personal sense of closeness."

Allisyn stopped. She looked back down, shook her head slowly, and took a deep breath.

Megan said nothing but embraced Allisyn's shoulder and gently pull her closer.

"We had an affair, Megs." Allisyn's voice was cracking, and she blinked away a tear. "I had an affair with Paul. While I was engaged to Jordan. . . . How could I do that, Megan? How could I possibly have done such a thing?" She looked up pleadingly at her niece.

"It's okay, Alli. I'm here. It's okay." Megan pulled her even closer.

Some passersby strolled through, averting their eyes and quickening their pace.

Allisyn slowly regained her composure. "It ended before the Nobel award ceremony, and Paul and I parted ways. He went to work in the private sector and ended up at Nu-Genomix. I returned to LA and took a premier academic research directorship close to where Jordan was living. We agreed to move forward and started discussing wedding plans. Except I never told him about the affair, even though I wanted to. I was so afraid of how he would react. I didn't trust whatever bond we had between us would be strong enough to overcome my transgression. So I simply didn't tell him...ever. I thought I could just bury it in my past, dismiss the affair as a minor indiscretion, a dalliance borne out of the stress and intimacy of the work Paul and I were both immersed in. And move on with my life. I sometimes think Jordan suspected it, but he never brought it up." She sniffled and uttered a soft, hollow laugh. "As if I could really forget it ever happened."

Now Megan's eyes were misting.

"So I just suppressed it. But the guilt and shame ate away at me inside and our relationship began to fall apart. Although I accepted full blame, it became harder as time went on to even consider telling him. We tried to make it work, but my failure to be honest with him and myself was self-destructive. Little by little, we began to grow apart and eventually agreed to break off the engagement. We tried to reconcile several times but just couldn't make it work. So I began doubting myself about everything. Could I ever trust my feelings again? I asked myself that same question over and over. Right about then, I was approached for the FDA position. Although I considered it attractive professionally, I also thought getting as far away from Jordan as I could would somehow ease the emotional pain and make it easier to move on. Foolish, I know, because those kinds of things never stop haunting you . . . never. We haven't spoken since."

Allisyn's eyes were dry now but slightly reddened. She closed them and slowly shook her head.

Megan gently lifted Allisyn's chin and looked into her eyes. "You can't beat yourself up, Alli. You just can't. It happened, and you regret it. But you have to move on."

"I've had a problem with trust in relationships ever since." Allisyn returned Megan's gaze with soulful eyes and the thinnest of smiles. "You have no idea how much having you here nearby, as infrequently as we get to see each other, has helped me through this. Just like when we were kids. I love you so much, Megs."

"Ditto. Wherever we end up, we'll always be there for each other, just like when we were kids."

They laughed softly together and embraced.

"Now you know the whole story," said Allisyn, having regained her composure. "And it's time you get back. I'll walk you over and catch a cab home from there."

"You know," said Megan as they were leaving the Quadrangle, "I can see how this little corner of the world could provide you solace. And I think I'll be back myself…often."

They both smiled.

CHAPTER

ELEVEN

"Welcome to the FDA, Mr. Krewe." Allisyn was meeting with Senator Gradison's chief of staff for the first time at his request. According to what his assistant told Ginger when scheduling, he wanted to get to know her a little better, since he hadn't previously spoken directly with her.

"What brings you here today?" she said.

"I was present for your report to the Senate HELP Committee, and both Senator Gradison and I are impressed with how you've reformed the FDA. So I thought it was about time I met you personally and relay the senator's high regard for the work you're doing there."

"Why, thank you. It's gratifying to know one's efforts are appreciated. Although I'm flattered and of course appreciative of his confidence in my leadership, I must emphasize it has truly been a team effort. Still, as much as we've accomplished, challenges still remain for the agency, both today and in the future, as I outlined in my written report."

"Of course. Let me be frank, Doctor. It's no secret the senator is considering a run for the presidency. Not to be presumptuous, but we're starting to think about the various agencies of the government and who should lead them under his administration if his presidential bid were to be successful. It's not an exaggeration to say he would like to see you continue in your position. Such being the case, I want to ask for your support of the senator in his bid for the presidency and gauge your interest in staying on as commissioner if he is elected."

Allisyn didn't exactly know how to respond to his premature pronouncement coming out of nowhere. She changed the subject. "Was there anything specific in my report you'd like to discuss?"

Krewe ignored her non-response to his probe. "Since you ask, one aspect of your report really caught the senator's attention. He's not scientifically inclined at all, nor am I, actually. But he was fascinated by your discussion of gene therapy and its potential in providing treatment for patients who are now being treated ineffectively or not at all. As you just alluded to, your written report to the committee addressed some future challenges for the FDA, including making sure new treatments like the gene therapy you mentioned are properly evaluated. I assume you include support for timely review of innovative therapies to avoid delays in making them available to patients. After all, our constituents are certainly expecting such action of us."

"Yes, indeed. However, our review process must be diligent enough to ensure they are not only effective but safe as well."

"Of course, of course. A good number of both senators and representatives, having reviewed your report, also reacted positively to the potential of gene therapy and seem to be supportive." Krewe paused and stroked his chin. "In fact, there is one particular treatment currently under FDA review which has received a good bit of attention. Apparently, it treats a specific disease which is somewhat common, genetically based and difficult to manage. You're familiar with it, correct?"

She frowned. *Ridiculous question.* "Yes, I am. The Nu-Genomix gene therapy for heart failure."

"Yes, exactly. I'm sorry. Of course you're familiar with it. It was foolish of me to even think otherwise." He cleared his throat. "It seems this specific therapy is getting a lot of press in the public domain, and those lawmakers have been receiving inquiries about it from constituents."

"Is that so?"

"I would imagine either they or a relative has the condition and would be a good candidate for the gene therapy if it were available. In any case, the inquiries are focusing on why the therapy approval is being delayed, and—"

"I'm sorry for interrupting, Mr. Krewe, but I must set the record straight on this." Her irritation index was rising rapidly. "The FDA has standard protocols for evaluating the safety and efficacy of new treatments such as the one you're referring to, whether it's gene therapy or something else. Clearly, these reviews must be complete and do take time. But there should be no confusion about it. There is no undue delay in this review."

"No, no. Of course not, Doctor. I'm not implying there is any intentional or even inadvertent delay. Apparently, the FDA's own Advisory Committee recommended expedited review of this treatment. Many are wondering why it isn't happening."

Allisyn thought how similar this conversation with Krewe was to the one she recently had with Secretary Vasquez. *Almost the identical verbiage, in fact.*

"If you're implying I, for any reason, am standing in the way of this approval, you are sadly mistaken . . . and to be frank, out of line. My role as commissioner is to ensure the safety, quality and integrity of the review and approval process and not introduce any undue bias one way or the other."

"Understood, Doctor. No disrespect intended. I don't want to be negative, so let me try to approach this a little differently. Perhaps we can look at it in a more positive light, one might say. Like the Advisory Committee did in recommending expedited review as a breakthrough treatment, I believe it's called. As I mentioned, you have Senator Gradison's support now and will in the future as long as he continues to have confidence in your ability to provide a valuable service to the public as FDA commissioner. As we see it, one of the basic, if not the most important, roles of whoever holds the position is to ensure timely introduction to the market of new and innovative treatment modalities needed by patients. Cutting edge treatments, if you will. If the president were to lose confidence in the process . . . well, let's simply say it wouldn't bode well for his continuing support of the FDA leadership."

He didn't say anything further, and Allisyn assumed the pause was intended for effect. In reality, however, no pause was necessary. Allisyn was now clear on the purpose of this meeting, and it seemed to align perfectly with the recent Vasquez discussion. Her head felt like it was in a vice, her face in a slow burn. She didn't trust what she might say, so she remained tight-lipped, letting him continue.

"Anything you can do to expedite the approval of the Nu-Genomix application would go a long way toward solidifying the senator's confidence and support in your ability to continue leading the agency in a progressive manner. I, for one, have the expectation you can find a way to retain his confidence by ensuring expedited approval of this treatment."

Allisyn wasn't sure if he had misspoken or if it was intentional, but she mentally noted his use of the word "approval" now, instead of "review."

His matter-of-fact way of bringing their discussion to a conclusion was not only appalling to Allisyn, but insulting as well. And the fact that he referred to the Nu-Genomix application specifically for the first time and spoke of expediting approval and not simply review left no question of what was happening here.

One thing was certain. She wasn't going to let herself be intimidated into doing anything inappropriate by what was political pressure at best—implied extortion at worst. But she needed time to figure out how to deal with the situation rather than debate the issue now. She was noncommittal, as she had been with Vasquez. "I'll think about it."

"Fine, but don't think too hard or too long. The Nu-Genomix team is extremely committed to getting their groundbreaking gene therapy to patients who can benefit from it as soon as possible. And they are pleased with Senator Gradison's support of their humanitarian goal as well. It's not likely they will let anything or anyone stand in their way. I'm confident you can figure out a way to retain the senator's confidence in your ability to provide positive leadership for the agency. It would be a shame to lose his confidence in your leadership, and I would imagine such a negative perception would follow you everywhere throughout your professional career. Thank you for your time today."

He stood to leave. As he approached the door, he stopped and turned to look back at her. "We look forward to hearing some good news soon from the FDA about this new era of successful gene therapy."

CHAPTER

TWELVE

Allisyn was sitting at the dining table in her condo, unable to stop thinking about Seth Krewe's recent attempt to pressure her into influencing the approval of the Nu-Genomix application. Taken alone, it was disturbing enough. But together with Constance Vasquez's previous meeting with the same intent and threatening tone, Allisyn's suspicions ratcheted up a couple of notches. *They're just too similar to be coincidental.* So was the proximate timing of their meetings, not to mention her phone conversation with Paul Westin prior to their conference.

Why? What do all three have in common in seeking the same objective? She dismissed Westin's attempt to influence her as an inappropriate ploy to leverage their prior working collaboration to advocate for his company's research under his direction.

But what about Krewe and Vasquez? She couldn't imagine what motive they could possibly share.

Struggling to decipher the common denominator between them, she ultimately settled on some sort of political power play she didn't yet understand. Which put her in an awkward and distressing bind, given her aversion to politics.

One thing she did know for sure, however, was she would have to tread lightly. If Krewe had accurately represented the resolve of the Nu-Genomix team in getting their therapy approved, she assumed they would go to any extreme to achieve their goal. Both Vasquez and Krewe alluded to potential adverse consequences for her if she didn't cooperate, which meant the possibility her career could also be in jeopardy was real. She needed help and would have to give some serious thought as to whom she might approach for it. *Definitely someone politically connected.*

Spending a little time on the semi-mindless task of straightening up her condo usually cleared her head. With this objective in mind, she brewed a cup of tea and turned on some mellow jazz music. Hopefully, she'd get lucky and come up with a plan.

As many people do, she had filed numerous papers and assorted documents she had accumulated over the years and moved them from place to place as she relocated. She rarely took the time to see if these long-neglected possessions were of any value, either materially or emotionally.

It was late in the evening when she came across a carton well suited for such a mundane task. Its label indicated it contained papers and notes from conferences she had attended, some of which were as a guest speaker. She figured she could discard some of the contents, since she knew only programs and the like were present. Her actual speaker notes and presentations were all cataloged digitally.

She broke the carton's seal, folded back the flaps and found what she mostly expected—conference programs, flyers and miscellaneous notes, most of which she readily tossed into a pile to be discarded.

When she came across a letter-sized white envelope marked simply "Contacts," she opened the clasp and removed the contents. As she sifted through the assortment of business cards and handwritten notes with names, email addresses and phone numbers, she realized these were all contacts she had made during a particular conference several years earlier at which she delivered a presentation on research regulations.

Halfway through the collection, she found a business card she recognized and came to a full stop. "How could I not have thought of this?" she said out loud while thumping her forehead with the palm of her hand. *Of course. It's where I met him.*

She silently chastised herself for forgetting the one person who would be best positioned to help her navigate the political morass she found herself in as a result of her conversations with Krewe and Vasquez. She resolved to correct the oversight first thing in the morning.

CHAPTER

THIRTEEN

It was just after noon the following day when Allisyn arrived at Carlton Gradison's office, having earlier spoken with his assistant to request an urgent meeting with him.

She found the senator standing at his assistant's desk, flipping through some papers. When he noticed his assistant looking up, he turned and saw Allisyn.

He glanced at his watch as he walked over to greet her. "Lunchtime," he said. "Have you eaten?"

"Uh, no," her eyebrows arching.

"Good. It's been one of those mornings, and I'd love to get out of the office, since it's such a nice day. Ever been to Eastern Market?"

She shrugged. "Guess I'm embarrassed to say I haven't ... even after two years here."

"Then you're in for a treat. Let's go. It's only a few blocks from here, it's a great day for a walk and my afternoon is open. You good?"

"Sure. Sounds wonderful."

After leaving his office in the Russell Senate Office Building, they casually strolled east through the tree-lined streets of the historic Capitol Hill neighborhood until they reached the Eastern Market, a 19th century brick building housing numerous markets and eateries.

Throughout the walk, their conversation vacillated between Gradison pointing out sites along the way and his complimentary remarks about her recent Congressional report and success in rehabilitating the FDA. He told her more than once how pleased he was to have recommended her for the position.

Allisyn had her own agenda for this meeting but was having a hard time breaking into what she felt was more like a soliloquy than a conversation. When they finally settled on a crepe stand inside the market for lunch, she wondered if she was ever going to get the opportunity to share her concerns with him about the meetings with Krewe and Vasquez.

"Now then," said Gradison after they had finished eating, "you wanted to meet with me. Sorry I got carried away. Let's walk back and you can tell me what's on your mind. My assistant said you referred to it as urgent."

Finally! "Are you familiar with Nu-Genomix, Senator?"

"The company you briefly referenced regarding a pending application for their gene therapy, right?"

"Mm-hmm, that's the one. Do you know anything specific about it?"

"No, other than the reference you made at the hearing. Should I?"

"Not necessarily." She proceeded to provide some background on the biotech firm and their pending application for the heart failure gene therapy. She referenced Paul Westin as a former research colleague as she provided some insight into the therapy.

"Now here's the thing," she said. "Our Scientific Advisory Committee thought enough of the therapy to recommend expedited review, considering it a potential breakthrough therapy."

"Meaning it'll be approved soon? A good thing, right?"

"Well, it was only a recommendation for expedited review. The CBER review team hasn't completed its evaluation yet, and they have the final say for or against approval."

"Hmm," he frowned. Reflecting on their conversation so far, she paused briefly then continued. "So here's what I wanted to discuss with you." She described her meeting with Constance Vasquez in detail. "She advised me to seriously consider getting involved in the review process and make sure the application was approved expeditiously. I reminded her the CBER Committee has the ultimate responsibility for approval or not, and our policy calls for a hands off approach from the commissioner."

"Why would she approach you with such a proposition?"

"Exactly what I'm trying to figure out. The only reason she hinted at was not wanting to resurrect any criticisms of overregulation by the agency as the cause of delays in approving needed treatments. Even though we recently discussed the need to follow our stringent protocol, she strongly advised me to intervene in getting it approved. And here's the worst part. She more than implied it would not bode well for the future of my career if I didn't oblige."

"I see. What did you tell her?"

"I didn't know what to say or how to react. I couldn't believe what she was suggesting. I told her I would think about it."

"So you're considering doing it? Urging the committee to approve the application?"

"Huh?" She thought she detected a sense of eagerness in his question. "I mean no, of course not. I just didn't want to get into a confrontational discussion with her. I have no intention of violating our policy."

"And did she accept your noncommittal answer?"

"No, not really. She said I'd better consider all the ramifications of not agreeing to what she was advising, indicating it would be in the best interest of my career to make sure it was approved. Which I really didn't appreciate."

"She actually threatened you?"

"Let's just say it seemed so to me at the time. Although I can't figure out why she would think it's such a good idea to even infer that. I suspected maybe she had a political motive, which is why I came to you."

Gradison looked away. "I don't know. . . . Can't think of what it might be."

She hesitated. "I had one more similar meeting you should know about."

"Really?"

"Your chief of staff also came to visit me. He said it was on your behalf."

Gradison stopped walking and looked at her sharply. "Seth Krewe? On my behalf?"

"Uh-huh."

"And what exactly do you mean by a similar meeting?"

She went on to describe Krewe's visit and how he attempted to apply similar pressure on her to approve the Nu-Genomix application.

"Hmm. Doesn't make sense."

They resumed walking.

"He said you were definitely in favor of fast-tracking application approvals for promising new treatments. And he cited the Nu-Genomix gene therapy as one such product. He went on to say how my getting it approved would really bolster your confidence in my ability to continue to lead the agency. Otherwise, he suggested, it was highly probable you would lose confidence in my leadership and ability to effectively run the FDA, and such perception could adversely affect my career going forward."

Gradison had been listening while looking straight ahead, and now he turned to face her. "That's not exactly accurate. I mean, yes, I do support the concept of removing unnecessary roadblocks to timely new treatment approvals in general, especially innovative treatments which hold real promise. Of course, it needs to be within the limits of appropriate regulatory oversight, as determined by your direction. But this new gene therapy? He referred to it specifically?"

"Mm-hmm. Sure did."

He frowned. "As I recall, we've never discussed the company or the therapy. Nor have I asked him to speak with you about it on my behalf. And I certainly would never so much as hint to him anything like what he suggested regarding the future of your career."

"I'm sorry, Senator, but it was clear his intent was to get me to intervene and ensure the treatment would be approved at your request. And if I didn't comply, it would jeopardize my keeping the position in your administration. If you were elected, of course. And such an outcome would be deleterious to my career. He made it perfectly clear."

He shook his head. "If I were elected? Outrageous."

They were about halfway back to the Russell Building and he stopped in his tracks. "Why would he approach you with such a threatening demand and say it was on my behalf?

"I was hoping you could tell me."

"Unfortunately, I have no idea why he would go to you with such a demand." He looked down. "Sorry you had to be subjected to such a bullying confrontation, Dr. McLoren. And by my chief of staff, of all people."

"I understand your alarm, and I'm sorry to have to bring it to your attention. It was so unexpected."

"No, I'm glad you did, as discouraging as it is to hear. Approaching you with such a request was out of line in the first place, and threatening you was bordering on extortion."

"I just want to know what's happening here. First Secretary Vasquez, then your chief of staff. Is there something political going on?"

He turned to her and shrugged. "I have no idea, Doctor, but rest assured I'm going to confront Seth and get to the bottom of it. . . . I can't even dream of what motive he and Secretary Vasquez could have in common."

She sighed. "I have to say both discussions were pretty disturbing. Besides the implied threat to me, knowledge of these kinds of discussions would resurrect unnecessary suspicions regarding bias in the FDA's review and approval process. And I don't believe any of us want to see such an allegation rear its ugly head again."

They stopped, having reached the entrance to the Russell Building. "No, we don't," he said. "Please accept my apologies for Mr. Krewe's behavior. I'll get back to you after I speak with him."

Allisyn thought of asking for a little more commitment from him in dealing with the situation quickly. Unfortunately, he didn't give her a chance. He turned and walked away briskly, putting his phone up to his ear.

"Have a good day," he said, waving his arm without looking back.

When she returned to her office, she checked her phone and saw there was a text message from Constance Vasquez: "Any update? Need to move this along!"

CHAPTER

FOURTEEN

When Gradison returned to his office, he immediately walked over to see his chief of staff. Krewe was on the phone and held up a finger as if to signal "just a minute."

The senator closed the door and took a seat.

When Krewe finished his call, he asked, "What's up, Carlton?"

"What do you know about Nu-Genomix?"

"The gene therapy biotech company?"

"Uh-huh."

"Only what I read in the FDA commissioner's report to the HELP Committee. Same information you got."

"Did you meet with Dr. McLoren to discuss the company in any way?"

Krewe hesitated. "Not directly. I mean, a little while after her report to the committee, I did make it a point to visit her. I never had a chance to sit and actually talk with her before then."

"Mm-hmm," nodded Gradison. "Go on."

"After her report to your committee, I thought it would be a good idea to get acquainted. I wanted to congratulate her on the great work she had been doing at the agency and thought I would take the opportunity to gauge her interest in staying on in your administration."

"My administration? A little premature, don't you think?" He didn't comment on Krewe's ignoring the question of whether or not he had spoken to Allisyn directly about Nu-Genomix or its product application.

"Possibly. I mean, I guess it is. But to be fair, it wasn't my main reason to meet with her. I only wanted to be sure she was aware you held her in pretty high regard in view of what she had accomplished thus far, and it seemed natural to see if she would be interested in staying on when, uh, if you were elected."

Gradison's eyes narrowed disapprovingly.

Krewe shrugged. "Sorry if I got ahead of the situation there."

"No problem. Although, like I said, maybe a little early in the process. Perhaps I'm more cautious on our chances of success than you are."

Krewe simply nodded.

Gradison looked away briefly, then back at Krewe. "Returning to your meeting with Dr. McLoren, did you specifically discuss the Nu-Genomix gene therapy application?"

Once again, Krewe was evasive. "Why do you ask?"

"There have been some rumblings among Senate members about their specific product application taking longer than expected to be approved. And Dr. McLoren might be getting pressure to move the process along to approval. I thought maybe it was why you wanted to discuss it with her."

"Pressure? Really? From whom?"

Gradison decided to pass on calling him out on pressuring Allisyn, at least for the moment. "Apparently, Constance Vasquez is anxious to have the application approved."

"Where'd you hear that?"

"Like I said, some chatter on the Senate floor. Any idea?"

"How would I know?" Krewe shifted in his chair. "If I had to guess, though, I'd say she wants to reinforce the appearance of the HHS secretary supporting the FDA's commitment to timely review and approval of new medical treatments. And the Nu-Genomix gene therapy certainly qualifies. Besides, as I recall, an advisory committee had already rendered a positive opinion on the treatment and recommended expedited review anyway."

"Makes sense." Gradison reverted to his previous question, pressing again for the answer Krewe had already sidestepped. "So when you met with Dr. McLoren, was the issue of their gene therapy application specifically discussed?"

Krewe shifted once again., this time sighing as he did. "As I recall, I believe we did talk briefly about the importance of new medical therapies being acted on expeditiously by the FDA so they can reach patients in need of them. Gene therapy was used as an example of a whole new category of treatments having such great potential and the importance of avoiding unnecessary delay in their evaluation and approval."

Evading the question again, thought Gradison. He was getting frustrated and more than a little irritated. "What about Nu-Genomix? Specifically," he said firmly.

Krewe began fidgeting in his chair and bouncing his knee up and down. He hesitated. "Uh ... I believe I may have asked if their product might be a case in point. Frankly, I don't know much about Nu-Genomix or gene therapy in general, actually. I was trying to relate what I had gleaned from her written report to engage in the conversation about the agency's approach to approving new therapies." He leaned back casually in his chair, seemingly more relaxed. "Why are you so concerned about Nu-Genomix anyway? As I said, my main purpose for meeting with her was to assess her interest in staying on in her role in the future."

"I was only wondering, when the subject of Nu-Genomix came up during the course of your meeting, if she herself might have mentioned or implied she was getting pressure to approve the application. Whether it be from Secretary Vasquez or anyone else."

Krewe started to fidget again. "Uh ... I hadn't thought about it before now. Maybe I wasn't exactly tuned in at the time, but I didn't get that impression from her at all."

At this point, Gradison figured it was about all he was going to get without a more direct approach. He straightened up, leaned forward and placed his elbows on Krewe's desk, inches from his face. "Dr. McLoren just met with me and told a very different story of your meeting with her."

Krewe pulled back his head, eyes wide. "Really? How so?"

"She said Secretary Vasquez tried to bully her into influencing the Nu-Genomix application, but she didn't know why."

"Funny. She didn't mention it to me."

Gradison glared at him, eyes narrowed. "What about you? Did you try to coerce her into influencing the approval of the application?"

Krewe didn't answer immediately, as if he was struggling with his response.

"Coerce?" he finally said. "I wouldn't go so far as to call it coercion. I just suggested their therapy seemed worthy of her . . . support. A little encouragement was all I intended."

"Just a little encouragement? Seriously?" There was an awkward pause. "Do you deny you suggested retaining her position as FDA commissioner if I was elected would depend on whether or not she made sure the application was approved? And that I would no longer have confidence in her to do her job if she didn't? And it would have deleterious effects on her career?"

"Not exactly. I—"

Gradison raised his voice a notch. "Not exactly? Again, yes or no?"

Krewe didn't answer, but instead just stared at him defiantly, his chin jutting out.

Gradison shook his head. "I'll take your non-response as a yes. What the hell were you thinking? That's outright extortion. What good could possibly come from it?"

Tight-lipped, Krewe leaned back in his chair and folded his arms. He stared at Gradison and hesitated before speaking. "For one thing, Nu-Genomix has a number of wealthy financial backers who were prepared to support your presidential campaign efforts and—"

"Are you telling me you tried to extort the FDA commissioner into ensuring approval of the application in return for some campaign contributions?" Gradison frowned, his back stiffening and his voice raising even further. "Have you gone mad? What a ridiculously foolish and dangerous, not to mention illegal, idea."

Krewe glowered back at him. "There's more to the story."

"Pardon me?"

"I was trying to protect you."

"Protect me? From what?"

"They had information on . . . questionable campaign contributions I had arranged as a lobbyist."

"You've got to be kidding. Campaign finance violations? Do you have any idea what a world of trouble we could both be in for?"

"It's why I had to do what they asked or they would make it public."

"Who's they?"

"I don't know. It was just this one guy who threatened me. He had a gun. Surprised me in my car. Said he would make it all public if I didn't get her to have the application approved. What could I do?"

"And he threatened you with a gun?"

"Not really. He just made it known he had one."

"What else?"

Krewe was fidgeting again and shifted in his chair. "Several of the contributions were for your earlier campaigns."

"Dammit, Seth." Gradison's face began to redden. "What the hell else have you been doing behind my back?" He looked away, shaking his head. "Illegal campaign contributions ... for me."

"I said questionable. It's a matter of opinion whether there was anything illegal about them. But your political adversaries would have a field day in the court of public opinion, and it would certainly derail your campaign, if not completely destroy your political career. And I wasn't going to let that happen."

Gradison leaned back in his chair, looking down, and didn't say a word.

"I was doing my job, as I always have," said Krewe, arms still crossed, now a smug look on his face. "Insulating you from anything negative. Plausible deniability. My only objective. He said it would never become public knowledge as long as I cooperated. All I had to do was get McLoren to make sure the therapy was quickly approved. I didn't see what harm it would do if the therapy was probably going to be approved anyway. I thought I could take care of it without getting you involved."

"You actually thought threatening and extorting the commissioner of a major federal agency was acceptable? Hell, it's not only unacceptable. It's criminal." Gradison paused briefly, looking away. "After all these years, I really thought you knew me better. You should have come to me about this, Seth. You should have come to me."

Krewe sat up straight, tense, hands tightly gripping the chair handles. "Come on, Carlton, you're a big boy. You've known all along how this game is played. There's always back-room dealings in politics. You simply never had the stomach for it. That was okay, though. It's what I was there for. You never asked me how I got things done."

Gradison brought his fist down hard on the desk. "Screw politics! Apparently, you think I need you for everything. There are a hell of a lot more important things in life than politics and political ambition. The only reason I even got into all this was because of you. Maybe that was a mistake."

"Stop being so damn self-righteous, Senator," Krewe said sarcastically, eyes wide like a trapped animal. "I never forced you to enter politics. I simply provided you the opportunity and support. The choice was yours, and you benefited from what I was able to do. It's always been me behind the scenes taking care of the nitty-gritty of promoting your successful political career. Of course you knew, but you never asked because you didn't want to know the details. And now you want to hang me out to dry for trying to protect you? Screw politics, my ass."

Gradison nodded his head. "We're done. This all ends. Right here, right now. The lies, the politics, the campaign. All of it."

Krewe looked at him with a blank stare, not saying a word.

Gradison's voice softened. "Doesn't matter now. What's important is you didn't trust me to handle the situation. Instead, you went along with their illicit plan and tried to extort the FDA commissioner. Which makes you complicit in a conspiracy, and I'm not sure the authorities will hold you harmless for your part in this whole mess, regardless of your intentions."

Krewe remained silent.

Gradison broke the silence. "I have to be honest with you, Seth. I have no idea how this will ultimately play out. And unfortunately, I can't imagine what I could do to lessen the impact on you as a result of your part in it. If you had come to me right from the start, it might be different. We could have fought this together. But now . . ." He rubbed his forehead between thumb and forefinger. "I'm going to ask you to take an indefinite leave of absence until this whole thing gets sorted out. I'm sure the FBI will be in touch given how you were threatened."

"Huh? Thanks a lot for sticking by me," Krewe said defiantly.

Gradison ignored the sarcasm. "Anything you can do to assist them will hopefully mitigate how they deal with your attempt to extort Dr. McLoren." He stood and turned as if to say something but just shook his head and walked out.

Krewe went over to the door and slammed it behind the senator as he left.

Gradison returned to his office and sat at his desk, critically assessing the confrontation he'd just completed with his chief of staff. Lips drawn tightly together, he stared out the window and nodded his head.

CHAPTER

FIFTEEN

Homicide Detective Hal Conyers' early morning flight from Baltimore to the Raleigh-Durham airport left him plenty of time to grab a rental and arrive at the Nu-Genomix campus in the RTP well in advance of his 11:00 a.m. appointment. He had called to speak with a representative from the biotech firm and was invited down for an in-person meeting.

As he approached the research complex, he was impressed by the expansive nature of the facility. The entrance of the main drive was flanked by a multi-stone wall about five feet high, with Nu-Genomix in bold gold lettering. The landscaping was meticulous. He followed the main drive and parked in the visitors' lot. The large steel and glass main building was imposing and attached to a smaller—but similarly designed—building to which visitors were directed by signage. Several small, non-connected buildings were scattered throughout the property.

The visitors' entrance to the attached smaller building led to a large semicircular lobby, which was equally dramatic. It had the look and feel more of a small museum than a lobby. The walls were adorned with numerous large-framed placards bearing various messages for visitors. Stories of the company's core research of genomics and various successful projects were bountiful. One wall consisted of a row of framed photographs of individuals associated with the organization, some in management and others key players in its research activities. Numerous chrome and leather seating options were scattered around the lobby, which was topped off with a cathedral ceiling highlighted by a large, segmented clear glass skylight. Two large video monitors with nearby seating were placed on separate walls portraying the story of Nu-Genomix and its work. Detailed attention was given to the current ongoing research around gene therapy. CEO Julian Shawe, Director of Research Dr. Paul Westin and numerous research personnel were highlighted during the fifteen-minute videos running on continuous loops.

After checking in at the desk, Conyers had enough time to wander around the lobby and absorb the various informational presentations before a receptionist approached him.

"Detective Conyers?" said the attractive young woman with an ebullient smile.

Conyers acknowledged her and was escorted to a small conference room next to what appeared to be an executive suite.

"Mr. Gardener will be in shortly," she said before leaving him.

It was barely five minutes before the door opened and a tall gentleman with reddish-brown hair entered. He walked right over and introduced himself. "I'm Bryce Gardener, laboratory operations manager here at Nu-Genomix."

Although not directly involved in the research activity, Gardener oversaw all operations of the facility, including staffing, supplies and keeping the place running smoothly.

The Detective nodded. "Hal Conyers of the Baltimore Police Homicide Department."

Gardener raised an eyebrow. "What can I do for you, Detective?"

"Thank you for taking the time to meet with me." Conyers sat at a small conference table opposite Gardener. "I was hoping to obtain some information about one of your research programs specifically related to the deaths of three of your participants. Trying to tie up some loose ends."

Gardener frowned. "I see. I'm happy to provide what information I can, Detective, but I must advise you it may be quite limited for reasons of confidentiality. Can you be a little more specific?"

"Understood. It's probably simplest if I explain how I came to learn of these individuals."

"Go on, then."

"It started out with my investigation of a friendly get-together turned violent and deadly. Two couples were out to dinner together, something they did often. The two guys were longtime best friends. So they were sitting there, the two wives carrying on one discussion and the two men their own. According to witnesses, including the wives, one of the guys just stopped talking and stared at the other for a brief period, then jumped across the table and started violently choking his friend. Other patrons tried to stop him but couldn't."

"My god! The guy choked his friend to death?"

"Actually, the guy being choked was about to pass out when he grabbed a knife off the table and stabbed his friend in the neck. Bled out and died right there before they could do anything."

"Interesting, not to mention tragic. The perpetrator ended up being the victim. Quite a twist."

"Yeah. Except murder charges were never filed. Not even manslaughter. It was considered self-defense."

"Hmm. Did he say something to provoke his friend, insult his wife or something?"

"Not according to the wives or other witnesses. Apparently, it was a normal, calm conversation until the original assailant just stopped talking and kind of zoned out or something. Everyone that saw what was happening said the guy had some kind of a blank stare like he was in a trance before he attacked his friend."

"And what does this terrible event have to do with Nu-Genomix?"

"One of the men was a participant in your heart failure study."

"Which one?"

"The deceased."

"I see. You mentioned something about three individuals?"

"Yes. I thought the description of his behavior just before he attacked his friend was so bizarre that I did some research, looking for deaths related to something similar. It wasn't easy, but I found two other incidents. Not violent altercations, but the part about the odd behavior that preceded their deaths—the blank stare."

"Hmm." Gardener scratched his cheek with a finger.

"The first was a tragic auto accident fatality. A man was driving down a New Jersey highway approaching a toll booth without changing speed. His wife started telling him to slow down, but he didn't respond. Never even gave any indication he heard her. She started yelling at him but still no response. Crashed into the cement wall next to the toll booth doin' about sixty. Killed instantly. She survived but was severely injured."

"Heart attack?" said Gardener.

Conyers pursed his lips and shook his head. "The autopsy didn't reveal any signs of a heart attack. And when the wife recovered, she insisted he was perfectly fine right before this all happened. He didn't complain of any chest pain, shortness of breath or other heart-related symptoms. What she did notice, however, was a couple of minutes before the accident, he stopped talking. He was staring straight ahead, eyes open with a blank look, not responding to her pleas to slow down."

"Like the guy in the restaurant."

"Exactly."

Gardener shook his head. "Pretty weird. And the third?"

"Right. This guy was playing with his granddaughter at the beach on Cape Cod, Massachusetts. They recently had a spate of bad weather and the surf was pretty rough. So he was keeping her close in ankle deep water. For no obvious reason, he stopped paying any attention to his granddaughter. She started calling to him, but he didn't respond and—"

"Let me guess. He had a blank stare like the other two."

Conyers nodded. "According to the girl, he was staring straight ahead, just standing there and not moving or responding. The girl started pulling on his hand and imploring him to get out of the water. Still no response. At that point, she ran back to her mother, saying something was wrong with granddad. When the mother looked up, she saw the same thing. He was standing still with waves lapping at his knees, staring straight ahead. All of a sudden, he began walking straight out into the water, moving with alarming speed. She called for a lifeguard, but the man lost his footing, fell and was pulled under the water, apparently by a riptide. Despite the lifeguards responding quickly, they couldn't get there in time and he was sucked out. Body washed up on shore about an hour later."

There was a brief pause between them before Gardener spoke up. "All tragic deaths. Is that it?"

"Yeah. Except for one more thing they had in common. All three of these individuals were participants in your heart failure experiment."

"Clinical trial, Detective. We call such research a clinical trial. Experiment is reserved for animal studies."

"Sorry. Clinical trial."

"So how can we here at Nu-Genomix help you? This sounds like a rather unusual coincidence."

Conyers frowned . "I don't know. Sounds too unusual to be coincidence. I was wondering if their demise was somehow related to your clinical trial. Not necessarily their deaths but their strange behavior beforehand."

"Uh, I don't see how. Probably just random coincidence."

Conyers hesitated. "You're not a physician, right? I mean, no disrespect but could we get your research director to give an opinion?"

"None taken." Gardener sighed. "Okay. If you have their names, I can let our research director, Dr. Westin, take a look at their records and see what he thinks. But truthfully, I really don't think his opinion will be any different."

"Great. It's all here," said Conyers, holding up an envelope.

Gardener stood. "I'll call you after he's finished."

"Thanks." Conyers handed him the envelope and his business card before he left, feeling less than satisfied with the results of his visit.

———

"That's all pretty interesting," said Paul Westin. "But truthfully, I don't see the relevance of these patients to a police detective, especially a homicide detective."

Westin had spent the last forty-five minutes patiently listening to Gardener's description of the lab director's meeting earlier in the day with the detective.

"It's not exactly clear to me either," said Gardener. "The only criminal investigation he was involved in was the crazy altercation in a restaurant where one guy killed another, supposedly his best friend. He didn't explain exactly how he came to learn of the other two individuals, even though he was trying to make the case all three were related in some way because each exhibited the same kind of weird behavior. And when he discovered all of them were enrolled in our study, he thought he found the connection. Along with the weird, trance-like behavior he described. Said something about tying up loose ends. Didn't elaborate any further."

"Mm-hmm." Westin twisted his pursed lips to one side. "Not very convincing."

"Agreed. Sounded like a pretty big stretch to me too."

"And how did you leave off with him? Is he going to continue bothering us?"

"Well, I had to admit I didn't have any medical expertise and would have to check with you. Said I'd let him know whether or not you felt there was any merit to pursuing this further."

Up till now, Westin had been sitting up straight, hands folded and resting on his desk. He leaned back in his chair, relaxed, and folded his arms casually across his chest.

"Hmm. Tell you what I think, Bryce. For some odd reason, this detective gets emotionally involved in what clearly are pretty disturbing deaths, and he's trying to put some closure to them. Don't ask me why. Maybe it's something he struggles with emotionally on a personal basis. For a detective whose job it is to solve crimes, perhaps it's an admission of failure of sorts if he can't explain them. Unfortunately, I'm afraid there isn't anything we can help him with here."

"If you're right, that's a pretty weird obsession."

"I'd certainly say so." Westin paused, steepled his hands and continued. "The way I see it, the only connection among these individuals is they were participating in our heart failure treatment study. Even then, they were probably enrolled in different clinical study cohorts. I really can't see how their unfortunate demise, each in a different manner, has anything to do with their heart condition or participation in our study."

"What about this bizarre behavior thing he referred to?" said Gardener. "He said they acted like they were zoned out or in a trance. Kind of strange, don't you think?"

"Strange? Bizarre? Sure. Also pretty vague." Westin shrugged. "Besides, who knows what those who witnessed the events really observed anyway in all the confusion of the moment. No, I still think this may be nothing more than the proverbial grasping at straws to make some sense out of random, senseless tragedies. To be honest, I wouldn't waste any more of your time trying to figure this guy out. I think it's best you get back to him, let him know we discussed it, and explain to him there's nothing else we can add to what he already knows."

Gardener hesitated. "I think it would be helpful if I could tell him you reviewed the files on each of the patients to confirm your opinion."

"You do, huh? " Westin paused briefly, then sighed. "Okay, sure, I can do that today. I'll send you an email if I find anything of interest. If you don't hear from me by the end of day, I didn't and you can let him know. And that should be the end of it. Okay?"

Gardener stood to leave. "Fine. I can't say I disagree with your conclusion. Like you said, probably some odd obsession of his."

Westin nodded.

Gardener walked over to the door and before leaving, he paused and looked back at Westin with a frown. "It just seemed he was so damn convinced there was something odd about this whole thing. I just wonder . . ."

CHAPTER

SIXTEEN

Bryce Gardener arrived at his office at the Nu-Genomix clinical research facility in RTP at his regular 7:00 a.m. time. He lived in a quiet, cozy neighborhood in a suburb of Raleigh, just a fifteen-minute drive to work.

He was thinking about his meeting with the police detective and subsequent follow-up with Paul Westin. Per instructions, he called the detective and advised him that Westin had reviewed the records of the three patients and concluded their deaths were not related to each other or their participation in the study. Still, Gardener couldn't stop thinking about the detective's dogged pursuit of an answer. What bothered him even more was Westin's seemingly out of hand dismissal of Conyers' conviction this was more than simple coincidence.

Despite Westin's opinion, Gardener decided to take a look at the records himself on the chance something might have been overlooked.

The detective had given him the names of the three patients, but the records weren't identified by name for patient confidentiality. Instead, the name of each study participant was assigned a unique number in a separate registration database. By accessing the registration database and using the names Conyers gave him, Gardener knew he should be able to identify their respective unique registration numbers and then locate their records.

But when he accessed the patient registration database, none of the three individuals were present. He double-checked the spelling of the patient names and had them all correct.

Odd. How was Westin able to review their records using their unique registration numbers if they weren't even in the registration database?

Frustrated, he was about to give up when he had an idea. He picked up his phone and dialed the number of Nate Burnes, a longtime buddy with a special expertise from their military days.

CHAPTER

SEVENTEEN

"Sure you wanna do this, Bryce?"

It was Saturday and the Nu-Genomix research facility was closed for the weekend. Using a special computer application, Nate Burnes had accessed the Nu-Genomix network and was about to disable the building's security cameras and alarm system without triggering any notification.

"Yeah," said Gardener with no hesitation.

Burnes had a background in military intelligence and operated his own IT and cybersecurity business. When he was first contacted by Gardener, Burnes warned his friend of the risk that others could potentially discover later what they were about to do.

Gardener insisted on going forward anyway.

Once Burnes was done, they entered through an employee entrance using Gardener's entry code. They went to his office, where Burnes sat at Gardener's desk and logged in to his computer. He plugged in a flash drive and started typing away while Gardener watched.

"Got it," said Burnes after about twenty minutes of tapping.

"The files?" said Gardener, jumping out of his chair.

"No. Not yet. But I did find a hidden drive like you thought, and it appears it does belong to your guy Westin. Odd thing, though. There's no password for the drive, although the data is encrypted. Guess whoever set this up felt the encryption was adequate enough. Getting at the data requires a decryption key, and that's usually pretty damn secure. Unfortunately for them, my little program I have here is running a decryption scan as we speak, and it may take a little time, but…" He paused for about a minute. "Never mind. It broke the encryption and I'm in the drive."

"Amazing. Pretty quick. How do you do that?"

Burnes laughed. "Here. Look at this. There are a number of folders, and I'm not sure what you're looking for."

Gardener scanned the list and fortunately, there were two of immediate interest. "Can you open these?" he asked, pointing at the screen.

"Sure."

Gardener stared intently at the screen, not saying a word.

Burnes waited a couple of minutes while Gardener scanned the contents. "I'm assuming you found what you were looking for?"

"Yeah, I think so. I'll have to review the files in more detail, though. There are some additional ones I wasn't expecting."

"So what exactly is in these files?"

"Some, uh, crucial data from one of our clinical trials that I couldn't locate. It's important I review it."

"Hmm." Burnes replaced the flash drive he used to crack the encryption and replaced it with another. "Tell you what. Let me copy the files you want onto this flash drive so I can close this down and get out of here. No telling whether there may be some alert process built into the drive's encryption. Unless you need something more, I think it best for us to move on out of here as quickly as possible."

"Uh, sure."

Burnes finished copying the files and removed the flash drive. He was about to exit the hidden drive and close down the computer when he paused and looked over toward Gardener.

He was across the room with his back turned, engaged in shuffling through some papers.

Without asking his friend, Burnes turned back to the computer and finished what he contemplated doing. He exited the hidden drive, logged off the network and shut down the computer. He walked over to Gardener and handed him the flash drive with the copied files. His hand on his friend's shoulder, he said, "Come on Bryce . . . now. Let's go."

———

Gardener slumped back in his chair, exhausted. It was well after midnight, and he had spent the last several hours at home reviewing the files Nate Burnes was able to access and download for him earlier in the evening.

He closed his eyes and sighed. He wasn't sure he understood everything . . . or even the significance of it. But he knew he needed to get this into the right hands. He just needed to figure out who that should be.

He went back to the files and began the laborious process of drafting a detailed summary of all the information present. When finished, he placed the printout in a blue folder, removed the flash drive from his laptop and hid it away for safekeeping. And he decided what to do.

CHAPTER

EIGHTEEN

Paul Westin stared out the window of his office while tapping a pencil on his desk. He couldn't stop thinking about his conversation with Bryce Gardener several days ago. A police detective had approached the lab manager with an inquiry about the unusual and untimely deaths of three individuals and if they could be related to their participation in the Nu-Genomix clinical trial for its new gene therapy to treat a particular form of heart failure.

Westin agreed to review the files of the three patients and advised Gardener to inform the detective that there was nothing to suggest their deaths were related to their underlying condition or participation in the study. What was bothering Westin now was that after he reviewed the files of each of the patients, his laboratory manager still didn't seem convinced by his assessment, noting the detective's persistence in pursuing the issue.

Ever since their initial conversation, Westin had been intermittently observing Gardener's behavior at work. He couldn't put his finger on it, but he thought Gardener seemed a little put off, distracted. Westin started wondering if Gardener had spoken with the detective again, and if so what he might have told him.

Westin decided to keep a close eye on Gardener. Having access to everyone's work email accounts as the company's research director, he logged into his computer and scanned Gardener's emails for anything unusual. The only one concerning him was made to the assistant lab operations manager at the Nu-Genomix Teaneck, New Jersey research facility, a fellow named Aldo Peroni. As Westin scanned the email, his suspicion was aroused when Gardener inquired about any irregularities or discrepancies in the preliminary animal studies forwarded to the Raleigh facility for inclusion in the FDA application. Since Peroni had responded that he hadn't noticed any, Westin initially dismissed the conversation as inconsequential. But the more he thought about it, putting it together with Gardener's apparent distraction after his interactions with the detective, he thought it would be better not to take any chances by overlooking anything, even if it appeared innocuous. So he continued to scan Gardener's emails and came across the confirmation for a recent airline reservation. The initial reservation was apparently made from Gardener's personal email. But for some reason, the confirmation was returned—or forwarded—to his work inbox.

Westin shook his head, picked up his cell phone and called a number. It was answered after two rings.

"We need to meet right away. There seems to be a problem."

"What's our urgent problem, Paul?" said Julian Shawe. He was meeting with Westin shortly after he received his phone call. Jason Tinley joined them in Shawe's office.

Westin briefed them on Gardener's meeting with the detective and his off the beaten path search for a connection between the three study patients and his own discussion with Gardener. He also described the details of the email exchange he discovered between Gardener and Peroni regarding the research project's preliminary animal studies.

"The more I thought about it, the more it bothered me," said Westin. "What if Gardener had some inkling there was more to the story and started snooping around our records? I started thinking we should check into things and see if we've had any data breaches."

"And?" asked Shawe.

"It appears our sequestered drive was recently accessed. The only other individual besides me who knows the decryption code is our IT director, and it was neither of us."

"Hmm." Shawe was drumming his fingers on his desk. "I thought your secret drive was encrypted and so well hidden. Our IT guy said it was undiscoverable and inaccessible."

"Yeah, well, apparently not as hidden or inaccessible as we thought." Westin leaned forward. "There's one other important piece of information from the log. We weren't hacked from outside the network. It was breached from within the network."

Shawe stopped the drumming and frowned. "This was done by someone here at Nu-Genomix?"

"Exactly."

"Do you know who it was?"

Westin hesitated. "It was accessed from Bryce Gardener's workstation."

"So it was Gardener."

"Seems so. Although it could be anybody using his computer if it was left on and unattended."

"How likely would that be?"

"Not likely at all. It had to be someone who knew or suspected there was a concealed drive in the first place. And based on Gardener's interaction with the detective and his email conversation with this Peroni guy, my bet is on him. Had to be. He was too fixated on the detective's story. Besides, I can't think of anyone else who would suspect the drive was even there to begin with, never mind what might be on it."

Tinley spoke up. "If it was Gardener, he must have had IT help to unmask it and break the encryption."

Shawe nodded. "Okay, we can agree it was Gardener. So what was he looking for?"

"Piecing it all together," said Westin, "I'm guessing he went looking for the records of the patients himself, even though I told him I reviewed them and there was nothing of concern. Then got suspicious when he couldn't find them. How he even latched on to the idea of a hidden server drive, I don't know. Lucky guess?"

"Like I said," chimed in Tinley, "a tall order for a mere laboratory director."

"The bigger question," said Westin, "is why does he even care?"

"At this point," said Shaw, "why he's pursuing this doesn't really matter. What's important is we contain this data breach and prevent any further access to those files." He looked over at Tinley. "Jason?"

Tinley's only response was an affirmative nod.

Westin shrugged. "There's one more thing. Gardener flew up to Baltimore and back on the same day after the files were accessed. I found the airline reservation in his email."

"Baltimore?" said Tinley. "What's in Baltimore?"

Westin briefly hesitated. "Not what. Who. . . . The detective."

CHAPTER

NINETEEN

For the last six months, ever since the less than amicable divorce from his wife of eight years, Gardener's nights consisted of tossing and turning, interspersed with only brief fits of dozing off.

Last night was no exception. He returned from his day trip to Baltimore late in the evening and went right to bed. He awoke at 5:30 and tried to get back to sleep, with no luck. He brewed some coffee, made breakfast and tried to watch a weekend cable news channel. That didn't last long. It was making him even more anxious than he already was, so he turned it off. The weather was glorious, so he decided to get some exercise and fresh air.

He changed into his biking clothes and strapped his Trek touring bike to the car's trunk rack. He headed out for the twenty-minute drive to his favorite route along a country road up and down the side of a small hill outside the city. The road was on the edge of a rocky ridge overlooking the beautiful countryside below. The view was always spectacular.

He parked his car at a roadside stop at the bottom of the incline, removed his bike from the carrier and mounted it for the leisurely ascent up the hill. He frequently glanced away from the road to enjoy the landscape below the narrow bike lane and was feeling better already.

About ten minutes into his ride, as he was taking a sharp curve on the incline, he saw in his rearview mirror a black sedan some ways back . He stayed far to the right in the narrow bike lane close to the edge of the ridge and waved his hand to signal the driver of the accelerating car to pass. But as it pulled alongside Gardener, it slowed and kept pace with him, moving closer. As Gardener looked at the car getting perilously close, he was able to vaguely see the driver through the slightly tinted window. The only detail he could make out was the man's crew cut and turned up collar.

Once again, he waved the driver to pass. But the man simply glared at him with an odd, twisted smile and stayed abreast, continuing to inch closer. Gardener gingerly moved farther over in the bike lane, right to the edge of the ridge, until there was no more room to move . . .

Back in his apartment, his cell phone rang and went straight to voicemail.

CHAPTER

TWENTY

Allisyn was sitting at her office desk reading and returning emails. It was one of her least favorite aspects of the day, since the list seemed to be endless on a regular basis. It was a close second to returning phone calls.

Ginger poked her head in to say there was a Baltimore police detective on the phone. "He wouldn't give me any specific reason for the call. Only said he had some information to share. Want me to take his number for a callback?"

"Nah, I'll take it now. Wait. A police detective you say? What could he possibly want with me?"

Ginger shrugged. "Didn't say. His name is Conyers, Hal Conyers. He's on hold. I'll put him through in a sec if he's still there."

"Detective Conyers?" said Allisyn as she picked up the phone.

"Speaking."

"This is Dr. McLoren. Sorry to keep you waiting. What can I do for you?"

"I have some information regarding a review the FDA is currently undertaking that I think will be of interest to you."

"Really? Sounds mysterious. Can you tell me more?"

"Actually, I think it best if we speak in person."

"Can you at least give me some idea of the nature of the information you have to share? As you might guess, I'm quite interested in what a police detective has to discuss with me."

Immediately after the words left her mouth, Allisyn feared her request might be interpreted as an attempt at a brush-off.

"Homicide detective, Doctor."

"Well then, I'm even more curious."

"Of course. An associate, for want of a better word, has brought me some information which I think will be relevant to the Nu-Genomix application that is currently pending with the FDA."

Allisyn bolted upright in her chair as if she had received an electric shock. She hesitated before speaking, her brief silence deafening. "Nu-Genomix? What kind of information?"

"It's sort of sensitive and fairly complicated. I think it's best if we discuss it in person."

"Can you get down here first thing in the morning?" She was aware of the tenseness in her voice and suspected he probably did as well.

"Yes, I can make it. If you don't mind, I'd like to have someone else join us. He's in North Carolina, so he'll have to call in to our meeting when I get there. Would that be okay?"

"Of course, if you think it's necessary. Although I must say I'm getting more and more curious about this. In any case, please let my assistant know when you leave Baltimore so we have an idea what time you'll be arriving."

"Will do. And thank you, Dr. McLoren, for understanding my hesitancy to go into any detail over the phone. And for accommodating me so quickly."

"Certainly, Detective. I'll see you tomorrow."

After they disconnected, Allisyn leaned back in her chair, closed her eyes and took a deep breath. Although her mind was racing, she didn't know what to make of this cryptic conversation. But she sure was looking forward to the next morning.

CHAPTER

TWENTY-ONE

The following morning, Hal Conyers left his brick row house in the downtown Baltimore neighborhood of Federal Hill—not far from the Inner Harbor—early after stopping for coffee. The area was characterized by historic brick row homes similar to his and an eclectic mix of locally owned shops and restaurants.

Just before he left, he tried calling Bryce Gardener to let him know he was meeting with the FDA commissioner later in the morning and he would like to have him join in by conference call. The call went straight to voicemail. He was a little bit concerned since he hadn't heard from the lab manager since he'd flown to Baltimore and given Conyers a blue folder of important information about the patients the detective had inquired about.

He looked over at the blue folder on the car's passenger seat. If Gardener was correct, everything the commissioner needed was in those notes.

Traffic was unusually light as he crossed town, passing Orioles Park and Ravens Stadium to get on Route 95 South.

He continued down 95 to the Washington Beltway, which would take him to the Silver Spring exit. Once he arrived at the FDA Building and parked, he made his way through lobby security and on to the commissioner's office suite. He was greeted by her assistant.

"Have a seat," said Ginger as she escorted Conyers into Allisyn's personal office. "Dr. McLoren is just finishing up a briefing and will join you shortly. My desk is right outside the door, so give me a holler if you need something."

As Conyers waited, he strolled around the room, gazing at the various framed certificates and citations, which were the only articles adorning the room other than books on the shelf. He paused when he came to the framed Nobel Committee Citation on the wall behind her desk.

"Pretty cool, eh?" said Allisyn as she entered.

Stepping away from her desk, Conyers turned to face her. "I'm sorry. I wasn't snooping. It's just that—"

"Not to worry. Detective Conyers, I presume?"

"Yes."

She walked over to him and they shook hands.

"I was just going to say how impressive that certificate is. I've never seen one up close, or at all for that matter."

Allisyn smiled. "Most people haven't. To tell the truth, I have to look at it from time to time myself to make sure it's not a dream. Very humbling."

"Yeah, I guess it would be." Conyers turned and waved his hand around the room. "The rest of your decor must be the most unpretentious ever for a government official."

"Ouch. Actually, I'd rather not be considered a government official, bureaucrat or whatever."

"Sorry—again. But I really did mean it as a compliment."

She chuckled. "Compliment accepted. Let's sit and you can tell me about this information you have. I have to admit, my curiosity is really piqued."

"Let me start at the beginning," said Conyers. "It all began with a very unusual altercation resulting in the death of one individual a while back, which then led me to two other unusual deaths. . . ."

When he was finished describing the specifics surrounding the three deaths that led him to Bryce Gardner, Allisyn hesitated, contemplating what she'd just heard. "I appreciate the terrible situations you have to deal with in your job, Detective, but I thought you had information about Nu-Genomix. Was I mistaken?"

"Not at all. I'm getting to that."

"By the end of the day, I hope."

Conyers smirked and continued. "So here's the thing. Although none of the decedents knew each other or even lived near each other, they all had three things in common. The described trance-like stare before the event that led to their demise, a long history of heart failure, and each was enrolled in the Nu-Genomix heart failure gene therapy clinical trial currently under review by your FDA."

Allisyn frowned. "Hmm. That is a coincidence."

"I don't think it is, Doctor."

"I see. And your reason is?"

"I went to the Nu-Genomix facility in North Carolina and met with a lab operations manager by the name of Gardener and presented the same scenario. He spoke with the director of research, a Dr. Westin. Are you familiar with him?"

"Yes. . . . And what did he say?"

"I was told by this fella Gardener that Westin reviewed the records of the three individuals and told him to advise me he felt it was all just a coincidence and had nothing to do with their participation in the study."

"I see. And you don't buy that?"

"A little skeptical, maybe, but it seemed I was at a dead end."

"Was?"

"A short while after that visit, Gardener reached back out to me to say he had some new information for me and wanted to meet. He flew to Baltimore and gave me what he described as very disturbing information."

"How so?"

"Said he decided to review the patients' files himself, but they were nowhere to be found. Until he enlisted the help of a friend of his who is a computer expert of sorts, and he was able to locate them."

Allisyn's eyes narrowed. "Really?"

"Yeah. Apparently, they were sequestered on a hidden computer drive belonging to Westin."

"A sequestered drive? Are you saying this friend hacked their computer system?"

Conyers didn't respond.

"I'll take that as a yes. So what did these hidden files show?"

"I don't know the details. But according to Gardener, the gist of it all seems to be the research team was aware of this behavior issue and it wasn't coincidence. In fact, there were other patients in the study that exhibited the same behavior. And none of them were included in the application they submitted to the FDA."

"You can't be serious. That's falsification of the application. Do you have proof of that?"

Conyers held up the blue folder given to him by Gardener for Allisyn to see. "Gardener drafted a detailed summary. It's all in here. Pretty scientific, so I couldn't understand most of it or grasp what it all means." He handed it across the desk to Allisyn. "I'm sure this will mean more to you." He paused, checking a text he just received. "If you don't mind, I'm going to step out to check in with the precinct. Besides, you're going to need some time to review that document."

Allisyn didn't say a word, just took the folder from Conyers, opened it and started reading.

Conyers poked his head in about twenty minutes later.

Allisyn waved him in. "Have a seat. I'm just about done."

After continuing to read for several more minutes, she closed the folder and sighed.

"What do you think?" said Conyers.

"If this information is accurate, it's very disturbing. I'd have to speak with this lab manager for some clarification."

"I thought you would," said Conyers. "I called him several times already this morning to see if he could conference call in with us but just got his voicemail each time. I left messages to call me back as soon as possible. I tried again just now before I came back in and still nothing." He changed gears. "Could you explain what you just read, in English? You know, in layman's terms?"

"Sure. It's complicated, but I'll do my best. To start with, all three of these subjects were apparently showing modest improvement in their heart failure symptoms after the experimental gene therapy treatments. But then there was an abrupt cessation of study notes on different dates for each of them. The final study note in each record, attributed to a research assistant, was within several days after their respective deaths. Each note was only a brief description of the circumstances of their deaths, along with a notation their files were removed from the FDA application document for death unrelated to study. Interestingly, each patient had an associated addendum file with numerous entries all dated after the patient's death. Signed with the initials PW, Gardener added a notation that he assumed they were authored by Paul Westin."

Allisyn took a long drink of water and swallowed hard, then continued. "And here's the damning part. For each of the three patient records, Westin's notes contained references like 'similar behavioral abnormalities as the other subjects,' 'behavioral abnormalities consistent with neural dysfunction due to genetic mutation,' and 'behavior similar to rare forms of temporal lobe seizure of genetic origin.' What's even worse is a comment indicating their behavior was consistent with what was noted in the animal studies."

"Animal studies?" said Conyers. "What's that have to do with this?"

"Animal studies are done before human clinical trials. These comments seem to indicate there were similar findings in those preliminary animal experiments. Eight hundred animals were noted to have what were characterized as 'unanticipated and inexplicable aggressive, violent and nearly rabid behavior' during the study period following the introduction of the synthetic gene designed to correct the heart defect in the animals. And according to Gardener's notes, all eight hundred were on this hidden drive and excluded from the application document."

Conyers looked confused. "As I recall, there's also mention of nineteen other patients. What about them?"

Allisyn nodded. "Right. According to the records, none of them died. They were also removed from the study findings, although for a different reason. Each was described as 'inappropriate subject selection' with no further elaboration. What was consistent among all nineteen, however, was each had been reported as having exhibited increasing agitation and unusually aggressive, near-violent behavior not present prior to entering the study. And the observation that the behavior was similar, albeit less pronounced, to what was exhibited by the three deceased patients."

Allisyn crossed her arms and leaned back in her chair. "Are you positive all this data was never made available to the FDA review team?"

"Gardener was certain of it. He told me he thoroughly reviewed the application documents himself and none of it was included."

Allisyn looked away, silent for a moment, then looked back at him. "I must admit this all sounds pretty bizarre. The comments about neural dysfunction lead me to believe they were thinking these behavioral abnormalities were related to a form of seizure activity. Temporal lobe seizure, to be specific."

"Huh? I'm sorry. You lost me there."

"Right. It's a form of focal seizures affecting only the temporal lobe of the brain and are frequently preceded by an aura."

The detective shook his head. "Aura?"

"Medically speaking, it's a peculiar sensation preceding the appearance of more definitive symptoms representing the actual seizure. Auras can be like mini hallucinations and take many different forms, some of which involve sight, smell, hearing, or taste. They can have other manifestations as well, such as déjà vu, nausea . . . and motionless staring. As well as an altered ability to respond to others, including a phenomenon called dissociation, a series of reactions ranging from mild detachment from immediate surroundings to more severe detachment from one's physical experience. And they can experience emotions which are not appropriate to their actual situation at the time, including a sudden sense of unprovoked fear or anxiety, even anger."

Conyers frowned. "So what do you make of all this, Doctor?"

"Of course, we can't know for sure, but the behaviors of the three patients you identified certainly resemble some of what's been described in these research notes, meaning compatible with a temporal lobe seizure."

"And the violent acts? Are they part of the seizure too?"

She took a few seconds to mull it over. "I guess if they had this overwhelming sense of fear, anxiety or anger, I can see how the seizure might further manifest itself as an inappropriate acting out in response to the specific emotion. Instead of the involuntary convulsive body movements typical of generalized seizures, their inappropriate actions could be consistent with the kind of severe detachment from their physical and emotional reality I referred to. Sure sounds like a dissociation reaction to me."

"In other words," he said, "their blank stare was this aura thing, and their actions after that were the actual seizure part."

"A little simplistic maybe, but yes, you could say that." She stroked her chin. "Problem is, the odds these three individuals all had a pre-existing seizure disorder of the same type and exhibited a similar manifestation are likely pretty slim at best."

"Coincidence?" asked Conyers.

"Not what I'm thinking."

"Sorry, Doctor. I'm not sure I follow you."

She leaned forward. "There's a rare but well-known variant of temporal lobe seizure disorder caused by a genetic defect. Probably what's being referred to in the notations in these research files. Except the chances of all three having a seizure disorder due to the same spontaneous genetic defect and with nearly identical physical and behavioral manifestations are slim to none. Not to mention the other nineteen patients. That would put the odds in the astronomical range."

"Wait. Are you suggesting something caused the seizures? The gene therapy maybe?"

"Technically speaking, it's possible. It's something we call an off-target effect."

"Huh? Can you explain?"

"Sure. It's one of the problems with so-called editing of a gene. During the process, changes can occur in other unintended parts of the genome which could interfere with a previously normal biological system. In these cases, the area of the genome controlling neurologic function would likely be the site of the off-target effect."

Conyers looked confused, shaking his head. "Then why wouldn't it happen in all the patients who were treated?"

"Because when an off-target effect occurs, it does so randomly in some patients and not in others. Certainly not all. In the case of these patients, when it did occur, it could've resulted in the unintended consequence of artificially creating the same genetic defect present in the spontaneously occurring form of the seizure disorder. The resultant malfunctioning of the brain's neural pathways is what would lead to the abnormal behavior. As for the three patients you originally inquired about, the trance-like stare they exhibited could be considered an extreme form of the aberrant behavior I referred to as dissociation. And with horrific and tragic outcomes, although in different ways for each. Similar, albeit less serious, behavior was apparently noted in the other nineteen patients so affected. And also with the study animals."

"Are you certain what you've explained is actually what happened?"

"Certain? No. I'm saying it's the only logical and scientific conclusion I can make based on what I know so far. And the research team members' notes in the patient and animal study files appear to support my conclusion. At least it seems that's what they were thinking as well. In other words, the frequency of this happening in both their animal studies and human trials is much greater than would otherwise be expected randomly. Which leads me to believe this really is related to their synthetic gene process and not some other extraneous factor."

Conyers scowled. "I don't understand. If they saw this happening in both animals and humans, why didn't they go ahead and do further studies to refine the process and minimize or prevent it before submitting their application?"

Allisyn hesitated before speaking, her response measured and her tone somber. "You would think so. It would certainly make sense, at least from a scientific research perspective. Unfortunately, the simple answer to your question is additional studies could take years and further delay the approval. And since they wanted to get their treatment to market as soon as possible, most likely for financial reasons, they instead chose to ignore the complication and withhold it from the FDA, knowing full well the chances their application would be approved were essentially nonexistent if the review committee knew about it." She shook her head. "The really terrible part is that they would never have received approval to proceed with human clinical trials if the complication seen in animals had been disclosed."

"Isn't that some sort of violation of FDA policies?" asked Conyers.

"Absolutely. It's an intentional misrepresentation of their research by withholding data they clearly knew showed the treatment is not reliably safe. It's outright fraud, tantamount to defrauding the government itself. A federal crime." She paused, thinking about Westin urging her to expedite approval of the application. "I presume you have all the documentation to support these notes?"

"Uh . . . we have a problem there, Doctor. Unfortunately, I don't have a copy of the data files themselves. Gardener has them on a flash drive. He wanted to keep it secured for now, at least until I spoke with you."

"Do you think anyone else at Nu-Genomix is aware you have this information? Or if they suspect Gardener does?"

"Don't know. He hasn't expressed any concerns to me yet. The original files should still be on the hidden drive, since they were only copied."

"Maybe, but you can't be sure. I think it would be safe to assume that someone will find out sooner or later. I need that flash drive with those copied records as soon as possible. It's the evidence required to substantiate his notes." She held up the blue folder. "I can't take any action against their application based on this alone."

Conyers was about to say something when his cell phone rang. Looking at the screen, he said, "It's Gardener. Let me take it and we can put him on speaker to join in and see when we can get the files."

"Yes ...yes," said Conyers as he listened. A pause, then, "What?" His face had taken on a near ashen look. He just listened during a prolonged silence before he spoke. "Yes. So am I. Thank you." Then he disconnected the call.

He stared at his phone without saying a word.

"What is it?" said Allisyn.

"Gardener ... he's dead."

"What?"

"A biking accident."

"A biking accident? Who was that on the phone?"

"Gardener's sister. The police recovered his cell phone in his apartment, and they tracked her down through his contacts. She saw I had called several times and left messages, so she reached out to let me know."

"What happened?"

"She said they're not sure. He was an experienced biker and out on his favorite route. It's on the side of a small hill, and the bike path is close to the edge of the overlook, a pretty steep drop. Even so, she said he was familiar with the path and traveled it numerous times. She couldn't explain how, but he apparently went off the side and down a rocky embankment. He was spotted by a motorist who called the police. When rescue arrived, it was unfortunately too late. Apparently, he had significant head trauma along with multiple other injuries. She said they're still investigating and going to do an autopsy to see if he suffered some health event that caused him to lose control."

Allisyn closed her eyes momentarily and sighed. "I'm so sorry for this, Detective."

"Yeah, well, I'm not so sure I buy this was an accident,"

Allisyn looked at him silently.

"Seriously," he said. "Doesn't it seem too much of a coincidence? I mean, this guy hacks into their hidden files and uncovers this damaging data they were hiding from everyone. I'm sure their IT system is advanced enough for them to discover a breach. Then he makes this trip to Baltimore and meets with me, a police detective of all people. They've gotta assume he's figured out their scheme and could be about to blow it all up."

"Are you suggesting he was killed?"

"Mm-hmm. Why not? From what you just explained, they're playing for high stakes here."

"If you're correct, and I can't get a hard copy of those files, I'm at a distinct disadvantage in addressing this problem here at the FDA. All I have right now is an employee's written description of this information. And he's no longer alive to attest to it. I need the actual data."

"I'll contact the Raleigh police and see if they can get a warrant to search his apartment for the flash drive or any other hard evidence to corroborate his notes."

Conyers rose to leave. "Thanks for deciphering all of this. I'll be in touch." He turned and left, shaking his head.

CHAPTER

TWENTY-TWO

After Detective Conyers left, his discussion with Allisyn consumed her for the rest of the day. It was exhausting just thinking about it. If what she read in Gardener's notes could be substantiated by the actual files, this conspiracy to defraud the FDA would undermine the agency's integrity, striking deep at the heart of its mission to ensure the safety of the drugs and treatments provided to the American public.

When she finally arrived home to her condo, it was early evening. She took a long hot shower and slipped into some loose lounge clothes. She ate some leftover pizza and sat on her couch, looking out the large window with her favorite view. She sipped some wine as she reflected on the detective's story.

It was clear she needed to prevent approval of the Nu-Genomix gene therapy application and expose this conspiracy to defraud the agency. She also knew to accomplish that, it was imperative to get her hands on the actual data and not just the written summary the detective had provided.

And as far as I know, the only place I can find that data is on Gardener's flash drive.

She'd have to tread lightly, however, so as not to tip off those at Nu-Genomix responsible for this deception. Especially if Gardener's death wasn't accidental, as Conyers suspected.

Something else was still unclear, however. She assumed Paul Westin, as Nu-Genomix research director, must have been aware of the data and resulting fraudulent application, a scenario both disappointing and frightening to her.

Is it possible he was unaware of this fraudulent conspiracy? Unfortunately, his initials accompanying the incriminating notes in the records pretty much rendered that possibility questionable at best. As unlikely as it would be, however, she somehow hoped it was the case he didn't know. More than hoped. She needed to find out one way or the other.

And what about Krewe and Vasquez? What was with their attempts to pressure me to expedite approval of the application? Allisyn was still waiting for Senator Gradison to get back to her about his chief of staff, and it irritated her that she still hadn't heard from him.

As for Vasquez, her attempt to intimidate Allisyn remained an enigma to her. Recalling the secretary's comments about some inquiries she had received about possible delays in the review process, Allisyn's best guess was some type of self-serving political motive. *Or was it something else? Surely she wouldn't push for approval of the therapy if she knew about this complication. Or would she?*

Allisyn was exhausted. She finished the last of her wine and called it a night.

CHAPTER

TWENTY-THREE

Aldo Peroni left work from the Nu-Genomix animal lab facility in Teaneck at his usual time of 5:30. He had been thinking on and off about the email exchange between himself and Bryce Gardener. He couldn't figure out what had Gardener concerned about the number of animal studies sent over for the heart failure FDA application. Peroni was certain all was in order. He knew he had to just put it out of his mind.

Right now, his objective was to beat the crowds and get home at a reasonable hour. He often didn't get to his home in the Bronx until close to seven. The commute each way included a subway ride and a bus connection. Home was less than a fifteen-minute walk from the subway station in the Bronx.

All told, his commute usually took between sixty and ninety minutes, depending on the traffic and crowds. Today, it looked like it would be closer to the latter. Both legs of the commute were typically crowded on weekdays, but today was uncomfortably so. It wasn't a good omen when two buses passed up Peroni's stop for the ride to the Teaneck subway station. When he was finally able to board a bus for the fifteen-minute trip, he was crammed in with everyone else, standing room only. It brought back memories of crowded buses back in his native Rome. Except this was nothing compared to the pushing and shoving during those commutes.

As the bus slowed to a halt and the doors opened at the subway station, the typical pushing and squeezing to get out the door with the others precluded any movement other than a slow shuffling motion—arms somewhat restrained at one's side—with those also leaving and others attempting to move to let them out. This accentuated right at the bus door, when Aldo felt a brief but sharp stabbing sensation in his right hip. He turned his head but didn't see anything unusual. He wasn't able to move much anyhow.

He finally stepped off the bus and was hurriedly walking in the direction of the subway when he felt flushed and started sweating. He suddenly became acutely aware of his heart beating—no, pounding—in his chest, seeming to be much more rapidly than normal. He stopped walking when he became alarmingly short of breath. A sharp pain developed in his chest, a tightening sensation increasing like a vise closing down. His vision blurred and he became dizzy. The last thing he saw before he slipped to the ground and fell unconscious were the faces of those around him looking down at him, some shouting, "Help! Help!"

Only one man seemed disinterested. He had a crew cut and a turned-up collar and watched just long enough to see Peroni lose consciousness. He turned and dropped a brown plastic bag into a nearby trash basket. The bag contained a medicinal bone auto-injector with a rapid-fire needle. It was capable of penetrating bone and instilling a medication directly into the bone marrow, where it would be rapidly absorbed into the bloodstream. The device had been emptied of its supra-therapeutic doses of Digitalis and Epinephrine, together capable of causing the rapid onset of a lethal abnormal heart rhythm and fatal cardiac arrest in a matter of minutes.

The man walked away and dropped a pair of plastic gloves into a different trash receptacle.

Jason Tinley had a return flight to Charlotte to catch.

CHAPTER

TWENTY-FOUR

Allisyn had a full morning of meetings two days after her visit from Detective Conyers. She still had not heard back from him as to whether or not the Raleigh police had found the flash drive among Gardener's belongings and wasn't very optimistic she would. So she did her best to put it out of her mind for the time being, since she couldn't do anything without those files.

It was late in the afternoon by the time she reached her office. She settled into her desk chair to read emails and answer phone messages. The number of emails was typical, but there were only a few phone messages, all of which she recognized. Except one from a Clarissa Brenner.

Curious, she immediately dialed the number. It was answered after three rings.

"Hello?"

"This is Dr. Allisyn McLoren returning a Clarissa Brenner's call. Is this Ms. Brenner?"

"Yes. Thank you so much for returning my call, Doctor."

"Certainly. How can I help you?"

"I'm Bryce Gardener's sister and…"

Allisyn sat upright and jumped in, not letting her finish. "I'm so sorry for the tragic loss of your brother, Ms. Brenner."

"Yes, yes. So sad. Thank you for your thoughts. . . . When my brother died unexpectedly, the police gave me his cell phone. As I reviewed the list of phone calls, I noticed a Detective

Conyers, Hal Conyers, had called him several times and left messages about Bryce traveling to Baltimore for a meeting. So I called the detective to let him know about Bryce's biking accident."

"I know. I was with Detective Conyers when he received your call."

Clarissa started to resume speaking, but her voice caught and started to quaver. She paused briefly, then cleared her throat. "I'm sorry, Doctor. This is still difficult for me. Bryce and I were extremely close."

"Please don't apologize, Ms. Brenner. Take your time. I completely understand."

"Thank you. I've been going through Bryce's things, trying to decide what's important and what's not. It's been difficult and taken me some time. Anyway, he had left me a note with a key to his safe deposit box in Raleigh and said he had given the bank authorization allowing me access to the box. There were the usual contents you would find in one of these, but also a small envelope labeled with specific instructions if anything happened to him."

She paused briefly, and Allisyn could hear some sniffles before the woman went on. "The envelope contained a small, portable computer disk, something you can plug into a computer."

"Yes, I'm familiar with the device. It's a USB flash drive."

"There were also instructions for me to call Detective Conyers and make sure he gets the drive. When I contacted the detective, he gave me your number. He was certain you would want the drive as soon as possible and advised me to give it to you directly. Something about research and the FDA, but I don't know specifically what it is."

"No problem. I believe I do." Allisyn felt her heart racing. "We had discussed it earlier. Some information on his company's product application under review by the FDA."

"Oh, sounds important," Clarissa said with a steadier, more composed voice. "I'm glad I'm able to get it to you after he . . ."

Allisyn perceived shakiness in her voice once again. "I'm sorry, Ms. Brenner, I know this is difficult for you."

"It's okay. Do you want me to mail it to you?"

"Where do you live?"

"Ellicott City, Maryland. Just west of Baltimore."

"Actually, I'd prefer to come to you and pick it up so there's no risk of it getting lost. My office is in Silver Spring, so it's a short ride. I can be there first thing in the morning, say around ten. Okay with you?"

"Yes, that's fine."

"Besides, it would give me a chance to meet you. Perhaps you can share some of your favorite stories about Bryce."

Clarissa sniffled. "Oh, so thoughtful of you, Doctor."

"Ms. Brenner, it's important for you to know Bryce was trying to do something good, something to save many people from being needlessly harmed. And some bad people wanted to stop him from doing it."

"Do you mean his death may not have been an accident?"

Allisyn quietly sighed. "I'm afraid it's a real possibility. The police are looking into it." She heard more sniffling. "You'll be helping Bryce make the difference he knew was needed by providing this information he wanted us to have. You should be proud of him and yourself."

Clarissa was silent.

Before ending the call, Allisyn obtained Clarissa's address and said she would call and let her know when she was on her way.

Perhaps I caught a lucky break, unaware of the two clicks at the end of the call.

CHAPTER

TWENTY-FIVE

Clarissa Brenner returned from running some early morning errands the day after she spoke with Allisyn. She hoped to get them done before her visitor arrived. She parked her car in the driveway and walked alongside the garage to the door leading to the pantry. When she put her hand on the knob, the door pushed open.

Damn. I forgot to lock it again.

She closed the door behind her, entered the kitchen, and put a bag of groceries on the counter. She walked into the den and was startled to see a man sitting in a chair. He wore his hair in a crew cut, and his shirt collar was turned up. An end table beside him supported a phone, a lamp, and an assortment of framed pictures.

She stepped back. "W-w-what?" Unsteady, she leaned against the door frame. "Who are you? What are you doing here?"

"Please, Ms. Brenner, I mean you no harm. I represent a group of important people who need a favor of you."

"A favor?" Her voice was quavering, her mouth dry. "I'm calling the police." As her gaze turned to the phone on the table, she hesitated. *What's that next to the phone? A gun!*

"I wouldn't recommend it, Clarissa." He rested his hand on the gun without picking it up.

That's when she realized he was holding a framed picture of two children.

"By the way," he said when he saw her staring at the picture. "these are two wonderful looking children. Relatives, I presume. Grandchildren, perhaps?"

Her body stiffened and her eyes widened, her mouth and throat too dry to speak or even swallow.

"I'm sure you would do anything to keep them safe," he said.

Clarissa tried to move but stumbled backward, almost falling. She collapsed on the sofa opposite the intruder, tilted to one side, staring down.

"Please let me explain about the favor. It's really simple. Later today, someone is coming to retrieve a USB flash drive you have in your possession. I need to see the drive if you don't mind."

She looked at him, lips slightly parted. When their eyes met, he looked back down at the children's picture.

She didn't know what to do. "I-I—"

"Please, Clarissa, don't tell me you don't have the flash drive. It would not be an acceptable response." Legs crossed, he tapped the framed picture lightly on his thigh as he glared at her.

She continued to stare at him, speechless.

"Please get the drive, Ms. Brenner. Now."

The tone of his voice frightened Clarissa even more. She rose to her feet, unsteady. With a slow, shuffling gait, she walked over to a desk in a back corner of the room. She opened the desk drawer and picked up a small manila envelope with "Nu-Genomix" handwritten on it. She walked over and placed the envelope on the table without getting close to him, then returned to the sofa and looked down at her hands folded on her lap.

He put the children's picture back on the table. "Do you have a computer?"

Hand shaking, she motioned toward the desk.

He walked over and inserted the flash drive into the laptop, proceeding to review the contents. After several minutes, he removed the drive. "Are there any other copies?"

Clarissa was still looking down, shoulders hunched. She shook her head without saying a word.

"Good. I certainly don't want to find out otherwise later on. In which case I might have to pay your grandchildren a visit." He walked over to the sofa and stopped behind her.

Without looking up she shuddered, then started weeping.

He glanced briefly at the children's picture again, as if in thought. Tapping the flash drive in his hand, Tinley looked back down at Clarissa. . . .

CHAPTER

TWENTY-SIX

Allisyn left for Clarissa Brenner's home in Ellicott City at eight the next morning. It was a forty-five-minute drive from her office in Silver Spring, assuming the morning rush hour traffic had subsided.

She was about ten minutes away per her GPS when she used her phone's Bluetooth to call Clarissa and let her know she'd be there shortly. There was no answer. *Hope she didn't forget I was coming and went out.*

When she arrived, there was no parking on the street where Clarissa lived, so she had to drive around to find an open space. She finally eyed a spot on a side street a block and a half away. Once parked, she began walking and tried Clarissa's number once again. Still no answer.

She approached the house, a cozy looking bungalow painted white with blue framing. A large, stately oak tree shaded the front lawn and the walkway to the front door. A dark green sedan, maybe ten or more years old, was parked in the driveway at the side of the house.

So much for her not being home. At that moment, a sense of foreboding closed in around her.

She rang the doorbell, with no response after nearly a minute. She rang again. Nothing. *Perhaps she's hard of hearing.* She knocked hard on the door and waited.

Still nothing. She tried her phone once more. Again, no answer. Now she was worried.

The door was solid with no windows and was locked when she tried the doorknob. She walked over through some shrubbery to the front bay window and peered in. The view was obscured by an opaque, gauzy curtain but was partly open in the middle. She carefully stepped over to get a better view, taking care not to stomp on the flower bed. When she looked in, she gasped. A women was slumped over on her side on the couch, a pillow lying on the floor.

Allisyn gently rapped on the window, but there was no movement. She pulled out her phone and dialed 911 and provided a brief description of what she saw. She put her phone away and walked over to the driveway to look in the car. There was nothing unusual.

It was only a few minutes before she heard the sirens. The police arrived first, immediately followed by an ambulance. Allisyn explained the scenario and stood back as they gained forced entrance. She followed them in, stopping to watch the EMTs assess the woman. She wasn't moving and didn't seem to be breathing either.

As she continued watching the officers and EMTs working around the lifeless body, Allisyn had a thought. She took out her phone and searched for Conyers in her contacts. She stepped outside and dialed. When he answered after two rings, she described her conversation with Clarissa, what she found when she arrived at the house and the current situation with the first responders.

Conyers said he was familiar with the area and would be there in twenty minutes.

She went back inside and saw the EMTs talking between themselves. They were no longer working on the woman. One walked over to Allisyn. "Is she a relative, ma'am?"

"No. Uh, an acquaintance."

"Sorry, but she was gone when we got here. Not sure of the cause. Hopefully, the coroner will be able to say."

One of the two uniformed police officers walked over and asked the same question. She gave the same answer.

"An acquaintance?" he asked with a skeptical expression. He looked down and took out a little notepad and pen. "And your name?"

"Allisyn McLoren. Doctor Allisyn McLoren." She spelled her last name as he wrote it down.

He didn't look up, pen poised on his notepad. "And what brought you here today?"

She hesitated, pondering how much detail to provide. "I knew her brother, Bryce Gardener."

"Knew?"

"He recently died."

The officer stopped writing and raised his eyes to hers. "And what is—was—your connection with him?"

"He had some information he left for her to give to me."

"What kind of information?" He resumed his note-taking.

"Research data. He worked for a research firm."

He shifted his weight, looked up and stared at her.

She sighed. "Okay, okay. I'm the FDA commissioner." She showed him her government ID badge and handed him a business card. "Mr. Gardener was the lab director for a company called Nu-Genomix. He had some information pertinent to the company's application for approval of a new medical treatment, and he wanted to share it with me."

"Mm-hmm." He hesitated, then reached in his pocket with a gloved hand and removed a USB flash drive. "Could this be it? It was lying on the couch next to her hand."

Allisyn's eyes lit up. "Yes, could be. Can I have it?"

He smirked. "No, Doctor. It's evidence." He put the drive back in his pocket and looked down, resuming his note-taking.

"Evidence?"

He kept writing. "We're considering this women's death suspicious."

"Suspicious? For what?"

He stopped writing and gazed up at her without raising his head. "Possible homicide. We found some blood spots on the pillow lying next to her. Problem is, we can't find any marks on her where the blood could come from. We'll have to compare the blood DNA to hers. If it's not a match, it would suggest a struggle. Which makes this evidence."

Allisyn nodded. "Can I at least get a copy of the information on the drive?"

"Look," he huffed. "I—"

Just then, Conyers came through the door and the officer looked up quizzically.

"Hal Conyers, Baltimore City Homicide," he said, flashing his badge.

"How did you get wind of this?" asked the officer.

"I called him," said Allisyn.

The officer rolled his eyes at her and sighed. "And what's your connection with him?"

"We're, uh, sort of working together . . . on the death of her brother."

"I see." He turned to Conyers. "Can you confirm what she's saying?" cocking his head in Allisyn's direction.

"Uh-huh. Her brother died in a biking mishap, and it may not have been accidental."

"And where was that?"

"North Carolina."

"Really? And you're involved?" He shook his head. "This is getting way too complicated." He paused and turned toward Allisyn. "So here's what we're gonna do. This flash drive stays with me until forensics is done with it. It'll be checked for prints and scanned. After the process is completed, we'll see about getting you a copy. But we keep the original. It's the best I can do, Doctor."

"That's fine, Officer. As soon as possible, please."

He nodded and turned back to Conyers. "If this turns out to be the worst-case scenario, Detective, we're gonna have to talk with you some more."

"Understood."

The officer walked back over to rejoin his partner.

"Well, that was interesting," said Allisyn after he was gone.

Conyers just frowned.

The officer came back over a few minutes later. "Sorry, but forensics is here and you'll need to clear out. I'll get in touch with both of you as soon as I can."

Conyers looked at Allisyn, then back at him. "No problem."

They went out to the sidewalk. "Have you ever been to this neighborhood before?" said Conyers.

"Uh-uh. Looks nice, though."

"Come on. I'll take you on a quick tour."

They walked a couple of blocks downhill to a busy street lined by an array of shops and eateries on both sides.

"This is Main Street," he said, "demarcating the historic district, an old mill town dating back to the late 1700's."

They continued to stroll down the sloping street. "It lies in the valleys of two rivers. As a result, it's been plagued by a number of destructive floods over the years. But the inhabitants and shop owners are pretty resilient. They've rebuilt every time."

He pointed to a stone building on an adjacent incline. "Over there is the oldest surviving train station in the country, built in 1830 as the first terminus of the original B&O Railroad line."

Allisyn was soaking it all in. "Amazing. What a treasure. I mean, not just the railroad station. This whole place. So quaint. I'd be here pretty often if I lived nearby."

They stopped at a coffee shop, each grabbing a cup to go. They continued walking, occasionally stopping to peek in a shop window.

After a short while, they headed back toward their parked cars.

"Hope you don't mind my calling you to come down to Ms. Brenner's," said Allisyn. "I was feeling a little put off by the officer who responded, and I thought it would help to have you there. Although I think it may have just confused the matter." She paused briefly while they continued to walk. "What do you think of all this, Detective?"

"I gotta admit, it looks suspicious like the officer said. And he doesn't even know the whole story. This makes Gardener's death even more likely to be non-accidental as well. Think about it. He finds the data, makes a copy, they get wind of it, take him out, and retrieve his flash drive. Which reminds me. I need to check with the Raleigh police to see if they searched his apartment for a copy. Obviously, he was smart enough to leave a copy for his sister and instructions for who she should pass it on to."

"If this morning was all about the data," she said, "how'd they know she even had it? And how did they get there before me?"

"Hmm. The only thing I can think of is they, whoever they are, had her phone tapped and picked up your conversation with her."

"Or just coincidence, which I seriously doubt."

He nodded. "Good thing you weren't there at the same time."

Allisyn stopped walking and turned to him. "Wait a minute. If they were after the flash drive, why did the police find it on the couch next to her?"

"Hmm. Good point. Maybe the perp left the drive as a decoy."

"Decoy? For what purpose?"

"Don't know. But this keeps getting stranger all the time."

As they approached Clarissa's house, now taped off as a crime scene, Conyers stopped. "I'll follow up with local police for their forensics report and see if we can get the flash drive to you ASAP. I was also thinking, with Gardener's death and now his sister's, this looks like more than just defrauding the FDA but a criminal cover-up as well. Maybe it's time to get the FBI involved."

"Mm-hmm. Makes sense. I'll leave that to you while I work on reviewing whatever's on the flash drive when I get the copy. Hopefully, it has the missing data and I'll turn it over to our review team. If not, I don't know where to go next. I need those files to stop their application from going forward."

They walked at a faster pace to their respective cars in silence. Allisyn sat and watched Conyers drive off. She was thinking of how her optimistic anticipation had melted into abject disappointment. And then there was Clarissa Brenner . . .

She pulled away in a separate direction, slowly shaking her head.

CHAPTER

TWENTY-SEVEN

"Doctor McLoren?" said Conyers when Allisyn answered her phone. It was the day after Clarissa Brenner's unfortunate death.

"Hi, Detective. What's up?"

"Just heard from Baltimore forensics. Clarissa Brenner died of asphyxiation. They found some subtle signs of trauma in her facial structures, so the presumptive cause was intentional suffocation. Probably with the pillow lying next to her."

Allisyn let out a deep sigh. "How horrible. Poor woman had nothing to do with this. Just trying to follow her brother's wishes, and she got caught in the middle."

"Mm-hmm. It does tell us one thing, though. Gardener's death seems even more likely now than ever to have been intentional. They must have suspected him of having the data all along."

"What did the Raleigh police find when they went through his apartment?"

"I called when I returned to the precinct yesterday, but they still haven't gotten back to me. Guess I'll have to call again."

"What about the flash drive from Clarissa's? Any follow-up on it?"

"Right. For starters, it had only her fingerprints on it. They scanned it for viruses and malware and it was clean. They said there was a bunch of scientific stuff they didn't understand. They can send a copy over to you by police courier."

"Great. Let them know I'll be in my office and I'll come down to the lobby when they get here."

"Will do, Doctor."

"Detective?"

"Yeah?"

"Since we're going to be working together, it's Allisyn."

He chuckled. "Fine, and it's Hal."

"Deal."

A little more than an hour after Allisyn's call with Conyers, she received a call notifying her the police courier was in the building lobby. She hurried down to retrieve the flash drive and immediately returned to her office and sat at her desk.

She plugged the drive into her computer and proceeded to review its contents.

There were two folders. One was marked GT-X-Patients, the other GT-X-Animal Studies, as described in the notes Gardener had provided. Both the Animal and Patients folders contained multiple subfolders.

She started with the Animals folder. It held large amounts of data, mostly numerous notations about the positive effects of the treatments. But nothing else. No comments about abnormal animal behavior.

Disappointed, she turned to the Patients folder. It contained subfolders which were labeled with what were presumably patient names. Conyers' three patients were there, with comments reflecting they were responding positively to treatment. Then there was an additional, separate note for each of them individually.

Interesting, she thought, when finished reading the notes. The verbiage was identical for all of them. Each patient was removed from the study due to "death unrelated to the treatments, study not completed." Conspicuously absent for all three was any description of abnormal behavior remotely resembling what

Gardener had described in his summary. There was also no mention of the other nineteen patients Gardener had cited.

Allisyn retrieved the blue folder Gardener had provided to Conyers and removed his summary notes to confirm what she recalled. Clearly described was the abnormal seizure-like activity of each of the patients, as well as the additional nineteen, and the abnormal animal behavior observations.

"Damn," she said out loud, bringing her fist down hard on the table. *The flash drive recovered at Brenner's murder scene must be a decoy. Just like Conyers suggested.*

She immediately texted him about what she found.

He texted back: "No surprise."

CHAPTER

TWENTY-EIGHT

"Quite interesting," said Alondra Parkes, Deputy Special Agent in Charge for Science and Technology.

Parkes was accompanied by two other FBI Special Agents. They just nodded with straight faces in Conyers' direction.

They were sitting together at a conference table in the J. Edgar Hoover Building on Pennsylvania Avenue, the main FBI headquarters in Washington.

Conyers had just finished providing all the details of the FDA scenario, starting with how the Cliffden deadly altercation had led him to the two other deaths and the Nu-Genomix biotech firm, his interaction with Bryce Gardener and the suppressed research data, and his collaboration with Allisyn so far. He included details of the deaths of Gardener and his sister, Clarissa Brenner, including the DNA results of the small amount of blood on the pillow suspected of being used in her murder. It didn't match hers.

Parkes had a puzzled look. "How is it Dr. McLoren didn't come to us directly with this story?"

Conyers shrugged. "My guess is that without evidence—the actual research data in question, not just Gardener's handwritten notes—she didn't think she had reasonable cause to take the issue to the FDA review team. After all, as the commissioner, her main concern was for patient safety. Since the withheld data indicated a complication of the treatment posed a significant risk of patient harm, her primary focus was on preventing its approval for use. I don't believe the legal aspect of the fraudulent application was initially top of mind for her . . . up until now."

"How so?"

"It appears the deaths of Gardener and his sister were meant to prevent this data from reaching the review committee given the negative impact it would have on the therapy being approved. A real game changer."

"I see." Parkes leaned back in her chair. "So what we have here is a case of defrauding the FDA, a federal crime in itself, compounded by two suspected murders as part of a cover-up scheme." She gently chewed on her lower lip before continuing. "What about the flash drive you found at the woman's murder scene? Anything come of it?"

"Uh-uh. No prints except for hers. The police provided Dr. McLoren with a copy, but she said the only data it contained is what was in their application. All the bad results were absent."

"Did she really expect her assailant would leave the incriminating evidence?"

"I guess she was hoping it was another copy of Gardener's drive Ms. Brenner had that her assailant wasn't aware of." He leaned his head back and sighed. "Can you get a court order to subpoena Nu-Genomix to provide the data?"

"Eventually, yes. But right now, we need to gather more information and background evidence, including the actual data Gardener obtained. Handwritten notes by a dead man won't cut it. A subpoena might actually induce them to permanently dispose of the data and deny it ever existed in the first place. Hell, they might even claim it was a made-up tale by this guy Gardener. At the moment, they have no reason to believe anyone has it other than themselves. And we don't want them suspecting otherwise until we're ready to move in. If we issue subpoenas for the information now, it would definitely tip them off we're on to the broader conspiracy."

Parkes shot a glance over at the other agents across from her. They both remained silent but one offered a subtle nod.

"Yeah, sure makes sense," said Conyers. "How do you go forward with this?"

"We'll start by speaking with the Raleigh and Baltimore police about the status of their respective murder investigations." She paused. "Did you say the lab director who alerted you to this hidden data had some help discovering it on the company server?"

"Uh-huh. It was on an encrypted hidden server drive. A friend of his, some kind of IT specialist, was able to locate it. Sorry, though. I can't recall his name. Although I do remember Gardener saying he had been an intelligence officer in the military, I think."

"I see." Parkes pushed back her chair to stand. "Okay, then. We'll get started and most likely reach back out to you and Dr. McLoren to see how else you could both help. We'll be in touch."

Conyers started to leave the room, but the sound of a voice stopped him. "Detective Conyers?"

He turned as one of the other two agents with Parkes approached him.

"Got a minute?"

CHAPTER

TWENTY-NINE

Conyers looked at the screen on his ringing phone. Having put the FBI deputy special agent's number in his contacts, he answered the call. "Hello, Agent Parkes."

"Hi, Detective. Just wanted to give you a couple of updates. First, we spoke with the Raleigh police about Gardener. They couldn't say much about how his presumed accident occurred, given the condition of the bike and his body at the bottom of the rocky hill. And they didn't find any kind of flash drive or other documents relating to the research data you spoke about when they searched his apartment. Doesn't mean much, though."

"Why not?"

"The place was pretty trashed. My guess is whoever tore the place apart was searching for the same flash drive you're interested in. Unfortunately, if it was there, the intruder must have found it."

"What about a computer, a laptop? Did he have one?"

"Yeah. They scoured it pretty extensively and didn't find anything of relevance either. Certainly nothing resembling the research data you described."

Conyers frowned. "Which makes it even more likely his death was no accident. Whoever wanted the drive with the data wanted him out of the way too." He paused. "I do have a question about how Gardener and his IT friend acquired the data in the first place. Any legal concerns?"

"Not really. We ran it by the Attorney General's office, and they feel it was company study data. As lab operations manager, he would have unrestricted access to the information. Which means having IT support to locate and access the data even though it was on a hidden drive is not in itself illegal. Their opinion is he was just dealing with a technical issue. It falls under one of the exceptions to the old "fruit of the forbidden tree" doctrine."

"Huh."

"On the other hand, it's definitely problematic for whoever put the information there in the first place. Since the data would definitely have a negative impact on the therapy's approval chances and it was both excluded from their application and intentionally concealed from discovery, it's de facto evidence of the company's fraudulent intent to withhold information from the FDA."

"Hmm. Makes sense." He paused. "Any other updates?"

"Not yet. Still working on some background information. We won't take any action until we hear back from Dr. McLoren confirming she's been able to get her hands on the data and what actions the FDA will take with the application. They have their own legal counsel. Besides deciding whether or not to approve the application, they need to render a decision on the fraud aspect. Although it looks pretty clear from my perspective. We'll keep you posted."

"Thanks."

As soon as they disconnected, Conyers called Allisyn to update her on what he learned from Special Agent Parkes.

CHAPTER

THIRTY

The morning after Allisyn received Conyers' call with an update on the status of the FBI investigation, she sat in her office, once again ruminating on her conversations with Vasquez and Krewe. She still had no reasonable explanation for their respective behaviors, as similar as they were. And to make matters worse, she was irritated that Senator Gradison had not yet followed up with her regarding his proposed conversation with his chief of staff.

As far as Paul Westin was concerned, up until now she considered his attempt to pressure her into approving the application was related to his role with Nu-Genomix.

But then she started having second thoughts about that assumption as well. *What if he didn't know about the data being deleted? Is it even conceivable anyone would be able keep the data concealed from him?* It seemed unlikely, but if it were the case, it would have to be Shawe. And confronting Paul might actually be a positive. *Playing to his psyche and pride as a research scientist, perhaps I can align him with me as an ally rather than an adversary...*

A ridiculous idea, she immediately chided herself while shaking her head. *Don't let emotions and the past get in the way of reason, stupid. He's the director of research. Of course he knows!*

She was left with the decision of whether or not to confront Westin directly about the missing data and fraudulent application.

Her initial thought was it would be a risky proposition to confirm her knowledge of the data's existence. It could trigger any number of adverse actions on the part of Nu-Genomix, including a preemptive permanent destruction of the data. And without hard copies as proof, she had no chance of credibly asserting an intentional fraud conspiracy. *Not to mention what those in charge at Nu-Genomix might consider doing to me personally.* A shiver rippled through her as she recalled the fate of Gardener and Clarissa Brenner.

She sighed. *He has to know.* Which would obviously mean, she concluded, he's complicit in the subterfuge, and it was unlikely he would turn against the firm. And to claim the entire scenario was an inadvertent omission was even less credible.

Whether he didn't know or—much more likely—he did, confronting him would be a precarious gambit for her and not an encounter she looked forward to.

She played every scenario of such a discussion with Westin back and forth in her mind. In the end, she was convinced she needed to meet with him despite how much she dreaded it. She immediately called him to set up a meeting.

"Paul, I'd like to meet with you as quickly as possible," she said after a curt, businesslike greeting. "How soon can you be available?"

"What's up, Allisyn?"

"We need to talk."

"I'm free now."

"No, I want to do this face to face. Where are you and when can you get here to D.C.?"

"I'm in Charlotte. The company jet can get me there first thing in the morning. Can't you at least give me a hint what this is about?"

"I've already said no. I can't. But it's important. Noon tomorrow in my office. See you then." And she hung up.

Elbows on her desk, Allisyn put her head down between her hands.

As promised, Westin was right on time the next day. "Do you have some good news for me about our application?"

"Not exactly." Allisyn got right to the point. "What do you know about some research data withheld from the documents you submitted?"

"Huh?" he said with raised eyebrows. He paused briefly, reassuming a straight face. "I don't know what you're talking about, Allisyn. Our application was complete. What data are you referring to?"

"There's reason to believe some problematic findings in your research were not included, findings which would definitely have negative implications for approval of your therapy."

He clenched his jaw indignantly and scowled. "What findings? Where did you hear this?"

Allisyn was wondering—*hoping?*—if her former colleague was truly not aware of the negative findings highlighted in the files.

"Let's just say it was brought to my attention some adverse findings from your studies were omitted from the application documents."

Westin did not respond immediately. When he did, his demeanor had softened considerably. "Oh, right. You know as well as I do some preliminary data is often excluded because of faulty collection and participant bias. Those findings are simply not credible according to the study design and would inappropriately skew interpretation of the overall data."

"Unfortunately, what you're describing is not the kind of data I'm referring to. And it includes both animal lab studies and human clinical trial data."

Westin leaned back, crossed his legs, and folded his arms. "Any kind of information you may have received from outside our organization is not legitimate, obviously fabricated by competitors to discredit our application and delay our approval."

She briefly contemplated how to respond to his misdirection. *Should I continue to play along or come right out and confront him with the data?* It wasn't a difficult decision. "Apparently, actual Nu-Genomix patient and laboratory animal research files exist, notated by your staff and in their possession, documenting a serious complication."

Westin tensed and didn't answer immediately. She presumed he was trying to think fast, probably because this was the last thing he expected to hear from her when they met.

"Simply not possible," he said with a smirk. His indignance had returned. "All our data is kept strictly confidential. No one could have access to it."

She knew he was now trapped. To claim ignorance of the information was to admit he had lost control of Nu-Genomix research oversight. To concede his knowledge of it was to admit complicity in its concealment and the conspiracy to submit a fraudulent application. She couldn't help ruing his predicament but nevertheless let his last comments hang out there without responding.

"Are you implying someone from within our organization gave you copies of this data?" he asked.

She didn't want to say too much and give away her hand. "As I said, the existence of such data was brought to my attention."

"Really? And what did this data specifically show?"

"Are you saying you don't know?"

He didn't respond, but simply stared at her. Assuming he would want confirmation of what the files contained, she proceeded to describe the pertinent details she had learned from Conyers by way of Gardener's notes. Specifically, she described the neurologic complication—severe, seizure-like behavior exhibited by a significant number of patients, behavior similar to what had also occurred in the animal studies. She gave no indication how she learned of this information. Nor did she suggest any files were in her possession. And she knew this was her vulnerability.

At first, Westin didn't respond, looking at her with a blank stare. She thought his silence indicated a non-verbal admission and indecision in how to reply. She was wrong.

"Let me see those files," he demanded.

Not having the actual data, Allisyn was unsure exactly how to respond. When deciding whether to confront him without the evidence, she feared it would be risky, since he could call her bluff and ask to see it. Now that fear had been realized. She responded by ignoring his demand and instead took a different approach.

She would make it personal.

"How could you condone withholding this information from your application, Paul? You must know the treatment complication you observed is serious, with enough prevalence in both animal and human subjects to question the safety of this therapy. As a scientist, what could you possibly have been thinking?"

Her ploy of misdirection worked, distracting him from his demand to see the files. "This is ground-breaking therapy, Allisyn. Do you know what good we can do? How this can be applied to other genetic disorders? Lives we can change, lives we can save? How can we accomplish any of it if we can't get this therapy into practical application?"

"What about the lives you're risking by not disclosing this complication?"

"Come on, Allisyn. You as much as anybody know all treatments have side effects. As innovators and researchers, we have to weigh the benefits against the risks. The history of medical research is replete with such compromises."

It was now clear to her not only did the data exist, but he was aware of it and complicit in the cover-up. Worse yet, he had rationalized dismissing this serious complication as simply a "compromise."

She felt the warmth in her face spreading. "What's happened to you, Paul? Have you been so blinded by corporate greed you've abandoned your professional ethos? You never thought this way when we worked together."

"Theoretical research is fine, Allisyn, but practical application is the end game. Organizations such as Nu-Genomix understand that, and those who push their innovations forward will succeed. If we wait for perfection, others will prevail instead."

Allysin felt her chest tighten. *I can't believe what I'm hearing.* This wasn't the person with whom she had shared intimate professional—and yes, even personal—moments of exhilaration. No, this was a different person, a person who could only be created by a single-minded organization such as Nu-Genomix, driven by power and greed—at any and all costs. She was both appalled and saddened at the same time.

There was an uncomfortable silence for what felt like an eternity before she responded. "I asked you here to understand if you were aware the findings of this research data were concealed. My intention was to offer you the opportunity to voluntarily take it to the review committee and allow you to carry on further research to refine the therapy and make it safer. I was hoping you would take such appropriate action informed by your research professionalism."

"What? You want us to pull the application and start over?" he said dismissively. "You can't possibly be serious."

"I see now you have no intention of agreeing to it." Her voice was resigned but firm. "In my capacity as FDA commissioner, it's my duty to ensure innovative treatments are supported and reach the public, yes. But not at the expense of patient safety. And I have no intention of disregarding such responsibility. Unless you agree to voluntarily withdraw the Nu-Genomix application immediately, I'll be bringing this to the attention of the committee and initiating suspension of the review process pending review of the absent data."

He leaned toward her, assuming a threatening posture, eyes narrowed. "Not wise on your part, Allisyn. It would be a mistake. A very big and dangerous mistake. I'm afraid it would trigger a series of untoward consequences for a number of individuals, not the least of which would be both of us. And for my part, I have absolutely no intention of allowing it to happen. As for the rest of the Nu-Genomix leadership, the investment they and other financial backers have made and their expectations for this reaching the market as soon as possible are too great for them to sit back and watch their investment dissolve. Believe me, these people will discredit you in ways you'd never dream of. Your career will be destroyed, if not worse."

"These people? And are you one of these people?"

"Don't be snide, Allisyn. It would be a grave error in judgment to underestimate what ends they'll go to in order to get what they want."

She felt the veins popping out in her neck and her head begin to throb. "Is that a threat?"

"I'm afraid it's more of a reality. Consider your professional career. All you've worked hard for and accomplished. The people we're talking about can destroy all of it. Everything. They have the resources to cast a pall on our work and make it easy to conclude our research together was equally tainted. Do you think the Nobel Committee would let our award stand with the knowledge of this information?"

Allisyn was fuming. "I don't care about any damned award."

He shrugged. "Perhaps they'll portray you as the aggrieved researcher whose work has been overshadowed by ours at Nu-Genomix. And that you fabricated this story simply to keep this company from succeeding in creating something you could not. How do you think such perception would affect your professional status? Would you be prepared for it?"

"I won't be blackmailed into overlooking this egregious act of scientific fraud," she blurted out in a raised voice.

"You're being foolish, Allisyn. They'll discredit everything you've ever accomplished, even the legitimacy of your current position. They can and will destroy your career and personal reputation."

She stood, body taut, fists clenched. "We're done. You can leave. Now."

"Don't be so rash. We should discuss this a little more when you're less agitated."

"Get out!" she shouted, throwing her arm up and pointing at the door. "Or I'll call security to escort you out."

"Think about it, Allisyn. We've both come too far to give it all up."

"Get out!"

As he left, she slammed the door behind him with her foot, her hands tightly balled into fists.

CHAPTER

THIRTY-ONE

"We have a problem," read the message.

Westin texted Shawe and Tinley immediately after he left Allisyn's office, requesting a meeting as soon as possible after his flight landed. They were waiting for him when he arrived at the Nu-Genomix corporate office.

"It seems McLoren has information about the research data we deleted from our FDA application," said Westin.

Shawe scowled. "Exactly what does she know?"

"Enough to delay or possibly terminate completely the review process. From what she told me, mostly everything we excluded. The twenty-two patients with neurologic issues, the three deaths and the preliminary animal studies."

"The only source of that information," said Shawe, "is in the records we sequestered on the hidden drive of the server, and only you and I can access them. It must be whoever recently hacked into the drive and has the data. And they must have had a good idea what they were looking for."

"Which brings us right back to Gardener," said Westin. "He must have told McLoren what he found. Had to be him." Westin started tapping a pencil on the table. "It'll be a disaster when he gets around to giving the actual data itself to McLoren and she—"

"It won't be a problem," said Shawe, waving his hand and dismissing Westin. He glanced over at his special assistant.

"I already took care of it," said Tinley. "Gardener's no longer an issue. And while I was at it, I thoroughly searched his apartment and retrieved a well-hidden USB flash drive containing all the deleted files."

"What if he made copies?" said Westin.

Tinley glanced over at Shawe. "That won't be a problem either."

Westin gave Tinley a quizzical look but didn't comment.

"I think it's very unlikely McLoren actually has any physical evidence of the data," said Tinley.

"You're probably right, Jason," said Shawe, "but we shouldn't take any chances." He turned to Westin. "What do you think, Paul? Since McLoren knew all the details, is it possible she has a copy of the files Gardener may have given to her?"

"Come to think of it, she only said the data which had been omitted from the application had been brought to her attention. Her exact words, actually, although she never said by whom. And she didn't even as much as imply she was in possession of any data or files when I asked her to show them to me. I'm certain if she did have an actual copy of the data, she would have made it known, especially when I denied it all."

"If Gardener told her," said Tinley, "how would he even know to go to McLoren in the first place?"

"Must have been the nosy detective who's been fishing around for information," said Westin. "Maybe Gardener told him, and he told McLoren."

"I'm confused," said Tinley. "Why would Gardener tell the detective?"

"Who knows," said Westin, shaking his head. "Right from the time he first came to me with the detective's goofy story, Gardener seemed preoccupied with it. For some reason, he must have bought into his idea about some connection between our study and the deaths."

"Huh. Weird if you ask me," said Tinley.

Westin turned to Shawe. "Whoever it was, they told her the specifics of what was in the files. She knew too much."

Shawe raised his hand to curtail any further discussion. "How she found out doesn't matter at this point. What's important now is she knows. Is there anyone else who might possibly know about the existence of the files? Even worse, what's in them?"

Westin shrugged. "Uh-uh. I can't think of anyone."

Shawe looked over to Tinley. "Jason?"

"Me neither." He paused. "Gardener does have—I should say had—a sister who lives in Maryland. A place called Ellicott City, just outside of Baltimore. She had a copy of the files, but I took care of them . . . and her too. Just in case."

Shawe nodded. Westin winced.

"However McLoren found out," said Shawe, "she knows too much. How was it she even shared this information with you anyway, Paul?"

"We met yesterday at her request. I was hoping to hear something positive about our application. Instead, she confronted me with her knowledge of the data. Said she wanted to give me the opportunity to voluntarily withdraw our application pending further studies we needed to do."

"Yeah, right," said Tinley. "As if that's going to happen."

Westin nodded. "She insinuated it might mitigate the consequences of our non-disclosure of the redacted files."

"And you told her exactly what?" asked Shawe.

Westin described how he told her the findings were only aberrant and not representative of the overall study results, that they were simply outliers because of several flaws in the initial study design, and the treatment overall had significantly positive value.

"Did she buy that?"

"No. She actually threatened to advise the review committee about the existence of the data and order an immediate cessation of the review process if we didn't voluntarily withdraw the application."

"What happens if she does take this to the review committee?" said Shawe.

"She'd probably invoke the Agency's AIP."

"What's that?"

"Application Integrity Policy. It gets the FDA offices of compliance, regulatory control, and legal counsel involved, something we definitely don't want."

Shawe stroked his chin. "Then what did you tell her?"

"That it wouldn't be a good idea for a variety of reasons. Especially for her."

"Mm-hmm. Well, we all know what's at stake for the company here. Our investors will not take kindly to rejection of our application, not to mention the potential scandal of collusion to withhold research data. If McLoren doesn't actually have hard copies of the files, then what she told you about them can only be considered hearsay and conjecture. Nevertheless, we can't even have her sharing what she thinks she knows, and we definitely can't let her get her hands on whatever files Gardener had. It's time we change the game and play our ace card."

Westin and Tinley looked at each other, then nodded in agreement.

"Well, then," said Shawe, "let's—"

"Wait," said Tinley. "There's one more loose end we need to take care of."

Shawe frowned and tilted his head slightly to one side. "Which is?"

"Seth Krewe, Gradison's chief of staff."

"What about him? He didn't help move the needle with McLoren either."

Tinley gave Shawe a smug look. "Word has it he's been placed on administrative leave."

"Who cares? He's no further use to us."

"True, but if McLoren contacted Gradison and told him about Krewe's attempt to strong-arm her into approving the application, then he likely also knows about Krewe's problem with campaign finance we used for leverage. The senator probably figured his chief of staff was damaged goods, and it would be best to cut any further ties with him to cover his own ass. I wouldn't even be surprised if he came out with a public statement denying any knowledge of Krewe's infractions and ultimately can him permanently. If you ask me, it would be the politically expedient thing to do."

Shawe shrugged. "Like I said, who cares? I still don't see how Krewe poses a problem for us at this point."

Westin was listening to this exchange between Shawe and his special assistant without offering any comments.

"Not necessarily," said Tinley. "Krewe's best play would be to go to the Feds for a deal in return for a tell-all on how we blackmailed him. It's what I would do if I were in his shoes. And it would certainly be a problem for us."

Shawe nodded. "Good point. Don't know why I didn't think of it. Then we should assume he'll do exactly as you suspect. How do you propose we handle the risk?"

"Eliminate it."

Shawe pushed his chair back from his desk and stood. "Then you have more work to do, Jason. And now I think we're done here."

After Westin and Tinley left his office, Shawe stood and walked over to one of the expansive side windows of his large corner office. It provided his favorite view of the beautiful surrounding landscape in the distance. He watched his special assistant in the parking lot below as he got into a black sedan with tinted windows and slowly drove off. He was thinking how Tinley had never failed him before.

CHAPTER

THIRTY-TWO

Allisyn was sitting at her desk reviewing a number of reports but kept getting distracted by thoughts of her conversation with Paul Westin about the Nu-Genomix application. She couldn't help fuming whenever it resurfaced. And the thought of how their Georgetown conference ended didn't help her mood either.

It was late in the afternoon, and Ginger was getting ready to leave for the day. She popped her head into Allisyn's office. "Need me for anything before I leave?"

"Don't think so. Only catching up on paperwork."

"Okay, then. I'm outta here." As she started to leave, she stopped and turned back toward Allisyn. "Oh, almost forgot. You got a phone call from a Phil Martinez. You know him?"

"Never even heard of him."

"He's one of those investigative reporters, and I'm using the term loosely. He reports for *People in the News Magazine.*"

"What's that?"

"One of those borderline trashy tabloids. You know, always publishing 'scoop' stories on celebrities, public figures and the like. Said he wanted to talk to you about someone."

"Name?"

"Didn't say. He insisted it was confidential. " She smirked. "And after all that gossip they publish? Huh, what a joke. Anyway, he left his number and asked you get back to him as soon as possible. It's in your message pile in case you decide to return his call. See ya tomorrow."

Immediately after Ginger left, Allisyn turned to her laptop and did a search for *People in the News Magazine.*

———————

When she arrived home early that evening, Allisyn decided to return the call from the reporter, as much as she dreaded doing it.

He answered after one ring. "Hello."

"Is this Mr. Martinez?"

"Yeah. Who's calling?"

"Dr. McLoren returning your call."

"Oh, great. Thanks for getting back to me so quickly, Doc. And you can call me Phil."

She didn't respond.

"Are you familiar with Amanda Leyfferts?" he said, not commenting on her silence.

Pretty direct, she thought. "Name sounds vaguely familiar, but I can't honestly say who she is."

"Co-host of *Today's Spotlight,* a daytime TV talk show with a mostly female audience. Sort of like *Oprah.*"

Again, she didn't reply. *Why did I even return this guy's call?*

"I have some inside information about a medical condition she reportedly has, and I thought you could provide a professional opinion on her problem."

Allisyn still didn't say a word, leaving another awkward silence, which Martinez broke. "Apparently, she's being treated for a number of skin cancers, and—"

"I don't think this is any of my business, Mr. Martinez. Or yours either, actually. Goodbye—"

"Wait, Doctor. As I see it, I'm a reporter, and people who read our magazine are interested in the lives of celebrities and other personalities in the news. They care about them."

Oh, please. Seriously? She was about to make a second attempt to end the call when he continued.

"Something called basal cell carcinoma, and I understand it can be an inherited condition. You know, passed on in the genes."

As annoying as she found this guy, Allisyn had to refrain from laughing out loud at his last comment. She just couldn't take much more of his nosy hearsay. "I'm sorry, Mr. Martinez, but I don't think I can be of any assistance to you. And if you don't mind—"

"I thought maybe we could meet to talk about this a little more."

I need to get rid of this intrusive gossipmonger, she thought with a sense of urgency. "As I said, Mr. Martinez, I'm afraid I can't help you. I don't make a habit of butting into the personal lives of others, even if it is a medical issue. Goodbye now." This time she succeeded in terminating the call.

She walked out to the kitchen to make herself a cup of tea, but decided on a glass of wine instead. *What a terrible job to have.*

CHAPTER

THIRTY-THREE

Odd, thought Seth Krewe as he stepped into the foyer of his house. *I never leave lights on when I'm not home.*

Krewe was returning to his renovated townhouse in Adams Morgan after eating dinner at a nearby brew pub. The trendy section of Northwest D.C. was located along 18th Street about a mile and a half from the White House. The neighborhood was known for its eclectic mix of residences, entertainment, and dining venues.

It was several days after he was placed on a forced leave of absence by Senator Gradison. Since then, all he could think about was how he had gotten himself into this mess and what was needed to get out of it. He wasn't looking forward to his scheduled meeting with an FBI agent the next day, but he knew he had no choice but to cooperate with authorities. It was the only way he had any chance of lessening the impact of his liability from the campaign finance problems and his part in attempting to extort Allisyn into approving the Nu-Genomix therapy.

Noticing the light spilling forth from his study, he walked in that direction and pulled up short at the doorway. There was a man sitting in the lounge chair off to the side of the large mahogany desk.

Krewe was startled. At first, he didn't recognize the man at all. Then he became vaguely familiar. When the man spoke, he suddenly realized he had heard that voice before and knew who it was.

"Sorry to surprise you, Mr. Krewe," said Jason Tinley. "We need to speak, and I couldn't chance reaching out to you in advance."

"W-w-what are you doing here?"

"You disappointed us, Seth. We really believed you would be able to use your power of persuasion to convince Dr. McLoren to approve the Nu-Genomix therapy. Didn't really think we would need to make your campaign finance indiscretions a public matter. But now . . ."

"I don't care what you do with the information at this point. The damage is done. Just go ahead and—"

"Make it public?" Tinley shook his head. "Regrettably, we're beyond that point, since you weren't able to get the commissioner to cooperate."

Krewe was quiet and started chewing on his lower lip.

"Oh, I'm sorry. I didn't ask if you ever figured out it was your friend, Connor Maxwell, who was helpful in providing the information to us. Doesn't matter now, though. Because it wasn't all he shared with me about you. It seems politics isn't the only interest you share with the ambitious legislator. Apparently, you're both fond of a particular form of recreation."

Krewe began shifting his weight from one foot to the other.

Tinley stood. "Unfortunately, your mutual habit is not only addicting but also can definitely be dangerous, even deadly, if you're not extremely careful. You see, nowadays, recreational drugs can be mixed with other potent drugs not routinely used for recreational purposes. Unfortunately, as I'm sure you're aware, such combinations can have tragic consequences."

Krewe's eyes were wide, his heart racing. He turned and headed for the door. Tinley reached him in two long steps and grabbed him from behind. Placing one forearm against his throat and the other hand on his head, he deftly turned Krewe's head, applying just the right amount of pressure as the man struggled in vain to free himself while not leaving any telltale marks on his skin. Krewe's efforts became weaker, and he passed out.

Tinley moved quickly now as he knew the effect of his maneuver would be temporary. He released his grip and lowered his victim to the floor. He removed the black leather gloves he was wearing and stuffed them in his pocket, replacing them with a plastic pair from the other pocket. He checked to confirm Krewe was still breathing and had a pulse. He dragged him over to the chair and pulled him up onto it in a sitting position. He rolled up the left sleeve of Krewe's shirt and placed a rubber tourniquet tightly around his arm above the elbow. He removed a syringe from his pocket and uncapped the needle. Easily identifying the bulging vein at the crook of Krewe's arm, he pierced the skin and deftly plunged the needle into the vein. He released the tourniquet and slowly emptied the contents of the syringe into Krewe's bloodstream.

He removed the needle and placed the syringe in Krewe's opposite hand. He carefully wrapped the unconscious man's fingers firmly around the barrel of the syringe, holding them there for several seconds. Then he draped Krewe's arm over the side of the chair and let the syringe fall to floor. After a minute, he raised Krewe's eyelids to be certain both pupils were nearly pinpoint.

Tinley removed the plastic gloves and slipped them into his pocket, replacing them on his hands with the black pair. Exiting the study, he paused at the entrance and looked back, the corners of his mouth turning up slightly. Then he exited the house through the same back door where he'd entered.

CHAPTER

THIRTY-FOUR

Carlton Gradison hurried back to his office in the Russell Senate Office Building from a committee meeting across the street.

He entered his office waiting room and immediately saw the visitor he was expecting. He walked over and introduced himself, extending his hand.

"Deputy Special Agent Alondra Parkes," she said as she stood up and flashed her FBI credentials. "Can we talk privately?"

"Certainly. In my office." Gradison told his assistant he didn't want to be disturbed.

"Have a seat," he said, closing the door. "What can I do for you?"

"Unfortunately, I have some disturbing news for you, Senator."

Gradison tilted his head and frowned.

"Your chief of staff, Seth Krewe, was found deceased in his home earlier today."

"What?" His jaw went slack. "You can't possibly . . . What happened?"

"He was to meet with me yesterday morning to discuss what he knew about an alleged conspiracy involving some biotech company and the FDA, as I understand it. He never showed. Two agents went to his home later in the day, but no one answered. They noticed a light on in one of the first floor rooms. Looking through the window, it appeared someone was sitting in a chair. They obtained an immediate warrant to enter the home and found Mr. Krewe sitting in the chair, unresponsive. Unfortunately, he couldn't be resuscitated."

Gradison felt the blood drain from his face. "Do you know what happened? Heart attack or something?"

"Not exactly. Initial toxicity testing showed extremely high—lethal, actually—blood levels of cocaine and fentanyl. And a syringe lying on the floor next to the chair held traces of the same."

"Someone killed him?"

"We don't think so. There was no evidence anyone else was there. His fingerprints were all over the syringe and were the only prints present. Unfortunately, all the evidence suggests he self-injected the drugs."

"What?"

Parkes hesitated. "To be honest, Senator, we suspect he intentionally overdosed."

"Intentionally overdosed? You think he committed suicide?"

"It could have been accidental, of course. But anyone regularly using cocaine would know the combination of those drugs used in the concentration present would surely produce lethal blood levels. So yes, we believe it was intentional."

"Wait a minute. You said regularly using cocaine. What do you mean?"

"Apparently, he'd been using cocaine recreationally on a routine basis. We found evidence of it throughout the home. You had no suspicion he was using?"

"Of course not. I had no idea. I would never tolerate drug use by my staff. But why suicide?"

"Perhaps he was despondent over his situation with the conspiracy and impending investigation of his role. Who knows what he was thinking?"

Gradison slumped in his chair, silently shaking his head.

"We'll continue to look into this as part of our overall investigation, Senator, and let you know if anything new turns up." She stood. "Again, I'm sorry to deliver this news. I'll see myself out."

After Parkes left, Gradison briefly looked out his window, then started reviewing and marking up notes from his committee meeting earlier in the day.

CHAPTER

THIRTY-FIVE

Not him again. Allisyn stared at the screen on her cell as it rang shortly after she arrived home. *I should block his number* She had just arrived home after a long day at work day and had no desire to speak with Martinez again. She just let it ring. Shortly after the ringing stopped, the voicemail icon showed up on the screen. Curiosity got the better of her, and she decided to listen to the message.

"Dr. McLoren, this is Phil Martinez. I really need to speak with you. I have some additional information I think you may find extremely interesting, to say the least. I'd appreciate a chance to speak with you again. This number is my cell. You can call me any time it's convenient, the sooner the better. Thanks."

She was determined not to call him back, and deleted his message. She picked up a medical journal to read in the hopes of taking her mind off the reporter. It worked until her cell rang forty-five minutes later. Her phone's caller ID again indicated it was Martinez. Frustrated at his persistence, she opted to answer this time and try to rid herself of him once and for all. *If I'm rude enough, perhaps he'll stop calling . . . I hope.*

"Hello, Mr. Martinez." Before allowing him to respond, she said, "I told you before the personal details and private lives of those individuals who are the subject of your reporting are none of my business. As I said, I don't believe I can be of any help to you, so I ask you don't—"

"Understood, Doctor. I appreciate your perspective on the merits of my profession—or lack thereof—and your reticence to engage with me. However, what I've come across transcends gossip . . . or a violation of privacy. Given your professional qualifications, I'm certain the information will be of particular interest to you. And if you give me a chance to explain, I believe you'll agree."

Resigned to the reality he was going to pester her indefinitely until she gave in and heard him out, she decided to get it over with. Besides, the sense of urgency in his voice now piqued her curiosity. "I'm listening."

"I'm sorry, but this is pretty sensitive, and I think we should discuss it in person. And the sooner the better."

She sighed. "I'm in Southwest D.C. How early can you be here in the morning? I have a busy day scheduled."

"Does 7:30 work?"

"That's fine. There's a little coffee shop, *The Beanery*, down at the waterfront. I'll meet you there"

"You're on. Oh, and thanks."

CHAPTER

THIRTY-SIX

When Allisyn arrived at *The Beanery* the following morning, a short walk from her condo, the early morning crowd had already started to dissipate. There were only a few patrons sitting alone, but only one was male. Before she could move in his direction, he stood up and waved her over to his table.

He recognized me, then thought it was reasonable to assume he checked out her bio on the FDA website.

When she reached the table, Martinez was still standing. He was wearing a blue blazer, unbuttoned, over a white dress shirt open at the collar, and casual khaki trousers. His hair was dark brown, full and slightly tousled.

Easy on the eyes, she thought, suppressing a smile.

He extended his hand. "It's a pleasure to finally meet you, Dr. McLoren." His voice was pleasantly casual, nothing like either of his phone calls.

As they sat down, he waved the waitress over, then looked at Allisyn. "Coffee? A pastry?"

"Coffee. Black, no sugar, please," she said to the waitress. "Nothing else. Thanks." She turned back to Martinez. "So what's this important information you have, and why do you think I would be interested in it?"

"Because in addition to FDA commissioner, you're the big kahuna in genomics."

Allisyn cringed, wondering where he was going with this. She didn't know if she could tolerate much of his flippant attitude or the kind of gossip he was apparently known for. She decided to play it straight. "Yes, my background is in genomic research."

"Ah, sort of like the work I do. Research, but a different kind."

She couldn't tell if he was serious or trying to be funny. She kept a straight face and didn't respond.

"Let me cut to the chase, Doctor. You remember what I shared with you about Amanda Leyfferts?"

"Yes, I do, but I don't see how I can help you."

"Let me ask you something first. Then I'll explain. . . . Is skin aging inherited?"

"What's that have to do with her skin cancer?"

"Humor me. Is it inherited?"

Allisyn sighed. "To say it's inherited is a little misleading. It's an inevitable part of the aging process for everyone. When it begins, and to what degree, however, can be genetically determined. So the short answer is yes, a strong family history can suggest a predisposition to early skin aging."

"Well, apparently Leyfferts has just such a family history and was developing early facial skin changes that didn't respond to traditional treatments. I guess a youthful appearance is considered important in her line of work as a television personality."

Allisyn smirked but didn't respond.

"She reportedly underwent an alternative treatment that worked extremely well in getting rid of the wrinkles, but then she developed the basal cell skin cancers. Is it accurate to say her particular form of skin cancer, basal cell carcinoma, can also be inherited?"

"Yes, but it's more likely to occur from a spontaneous or induced genetic mutation alone or coupled with environmental factors."

"Induced? By what?"

"Anything that causes a change in the portion of the gene that controls skin development. Like extreme radiation exposure or many years of excess exposure to the sun's rays. Even excess UV light exposure. . . . Was that her treatment?"

"No, but I'll get to that in a bit. First, let me tell you about two other individuals, both high-profile. Do you know who Kyle Apeloko is?"

"Isn't he the South African runner who's won a whole bunch of Olympic and World Cup marathon races?"

"Yeah and—"

"Immigrated to the States a while back, didn't he?"

"Right again. He moved here to take advantage of the financial benefits of his athletic success and notoriety. Problem is, his victories tailed off significantly. Likely from aging—less stamina than the youngsters. Unfortunately, it was detrimental to his financial prospects. I guess an athletic has-been doesn't get too many endorsement offers, and long-distance running isn't exactly good preparation for a business career."

Allisyn suddenly remembered something else. "Wait a minute. Didn't he recently die during a race? Collapsed in the middle of it?"

He nodded. "Now you're in the groove."

She rolled her eyes but otherwise ignored his comment. "Did they do an autopsy?"

"Of course."

"My guess is he had an MI. He was well along in age for such an activity, at least competitively. Or maybe a fatal arrhythmia, an erratic heartbeat."

Martinez looked askance at Allisyn. "I know what an arrhythmia is."

She felt her face warm and immediately regretted her comment. "What did they find?"

"Massive heart attack as you suggested. All his coronary arteries were completely blocked by blood clots."

"Pretty odd. Rather unusual, actually."

"What's even more unusual was his entire circulatory system was filled with clot-like sludge."

"Hmm. Some type of bizarre, disseminated coagulopathy, abnormal—"

"Blood clotting. I know, I know."

Allisyn hesitated, not wanting to offend him again. "You're pretty good with your medical knowledge and terminology."

"Like I said, research and reporting are what I do. When I come across a story with background I'm not familiar with, I make it my job to learn as much as I can about it."

"I'm impressed. Seriously."

He gave her an appreciative nod.

"Was he on any medication? Something which would perhaps cause clotting under unusual circumstances?"

"Uh-uh. WADA even considered the possibility of blood doping with PED. You know, performance enhancing drugs. But there was no evidence of steroids or other PED."

She weakly smiled at his need to define PED. "Okay, you got me there. What's WADA?"

"Sorry. The World Anti-Doping Agency. They monitor athletes around the world for the use of PED. They're the international equivalent of the U.S. Anti-Doping Agency. . . . There is one other substance they reportedly checked him for, something called EPO. Except it didn't show up."

Allisyn's eyes widened. "EPO is short for Erythropoietin, a protein which acts as a hormone controlling red blood cell production."

"Right. Apparently, athletes in the past have utilized blood doping by self-injecting this EPO protein to enhance their performance during an athletic competition."

"Makes sense." She explained how the additional EPO would increase the production of red blood cells in the circulation, thereby boosting the amount of oxygen available to muscle.

"Which in turn enhances an athlete's endurance and performance. And if the red blood cell production was way overstimulated—"

Martinez jumped in. "The blood would be thickened and result in excess clotting and sludging."

"Exactly. At least that's a possibility." It was obvious to Allisyn the reporter had indeed done his homework.

"But couldn't they test for the EPO protein in the blood?" he asked.

"Only if it was exogenous EPO, chemically manufactured outside the body and then injected into the bloodstream. Exactly what you described as blood doping with those athletes in the past. If it's produced within the body's own cells, however, it's not as distinctly identifiable as abnormal."

"So if the EPO was produced by his own body, does that mean you wouldn't consider the increased red cells a result of intentional blood doping?"

"Not necessarily. Depends on how his body came to produce the EPO excess in the first place."

"You mean if his body was stimulated in some artificial way to produce more of its own EPO to intentionally increase the red cell production. Is that even possible?"

"Theoretically, yes. Production of the protein is controlled by a specific gene, so—"

"What if there was an injection, or whatever you do, of that gene to stimulate the body's own production of EPO?"

"Again, theoretically possible. In which case I guess you would refer to it as gene doping, the genetic equivalent of performance enhancing drugs. Except I've never heard of that being done."

Martinez sighed. "Let me tell you about one other individual. Then we can talk about that a little more. Do you recognize the name Kaylie Edgers?"

"Sure. She's that highly successful tennis pro. Has multiple Grand Slam championships."

"Yep."

"Don't tell me she has some rare inherited disease . . . if that's where you're going with all this."

"No, not at all. But her daughter, Felicity, was recently diagnosed with an abdominal tumor, something called rhabdomyosarcoma."

Allisyn jerked her head and frowned. "That's terrible."

Martinez paused to sip his coffee, which had cooled off. He called the waitress over for two fresh cups.

"I'm sorry, Mr. Martinez, but how do you acquire this kind of information? After all, it is protected health care material."

"I have my sources, Doctor."

"I see." She was tempted to ask whether or not those sources were legal, but then thought better of it.

Undaunted, Martinez didn't address her concern any further. "About this rhabdo . . . whatever. Is it inherited?"

"Technically, no, but—"

"Which takes me to what I've learned about what these three individuals have in common."

Allisyn was growing weary of his habit of repeatedly finishing her sentences, or worse, outright interrupting her. But the reporter was clearly going somewhere with this, and she let it slide for now. "Go on. I'm listening."

"What if I told you all three had a particular medical treatment, a gene implant of some kind?"

"What? I'd say you're crazy, since such a procedure for non-therapeutic purposes hasn't yet been approved."

"Not here. But what about somewhere else? Another country?"

"And how would you know about it, since I don't?"

"Like I said, I have my sources and they're reliable and discrete, although not conventional in their methods. It's my job. Investigative reporting. As I said, research, much like you. Except I research people and their lives because it's what the public wants to hear about, whether it's good, bad or ugly. And for this kind of information, I need specialized sources."

"How admirable." She remained expressionless. *Probably has a network of hackers.*

"Regardless of your opinion of my, uh, profession, Doctor, I do serve a purpose. Fill a void for many people. Y'know?"

She suddenly remembered him saying something similar when they first spoke on the phone. Now she felt guilty but chose not to say anything about her sarcastic comment.

"Nothing like what you're talking about," she said, "is commercially available yet, certainly not approved by the FDA or even tested to my knowledge."

"Like I said, maybe not here in the States."

"Let me get this straight. You're suggesting some sort of gene therapy is being used outside this country for elective, non-therapeutic purposes?"

Martinez leaned forward, glancing right then left. "Have you ever heard of the Institute for Personal Enhancement, IPE?"

"Nope. Doesn't ring a bell."

"Not surprising, since it's tucked away in Malaysia."

"Malaysia? On the other side of the world? No wonder I've never heard of it."

"Yeah, that and the fact it's not a traditional medical facility. Probably why it hasn't shown up in your scientific journals. But it does exist. And my sources confirm all three—Apeloko, Leyfferts, and Felicity Edgers—received some form of gene therapy at the facility."

She shook her head. "Let me see if I follow you here. You're saying these three individuals—"

"And probably others."

"Okay, maybe others. But these three you've referred to presumably had a form of elective genetic manipulation at an obscure clinic, or so-called institute no one knows about in another country, for non-therapeutic enhancement purposes. And this facility doesn't show up in any traditional medical literature source. Yet individuals who are motivated enough can find out about it. Have I got it right?"

"Pretty much."

She shrugged. "Okay, let's say I buy into this scenario . . . for the time being. And I'm being generous here. Explain how Edgers' daughter and Leyfferts fit in."

He looked around again and lowered his voice. "My sources tell me Kaylie Edgers was grooming her daughter for a career in professional tennis like her. It's common knowledge Kaylie is an extremely driven individual, a fierce competitor. Her father, a tennis legend himself, pushed her hard growing up. And when her daughter was born, Kaylie had the same success in mind for Felicity. Despite all the best instruction and physical trainers, however, Felicity didn't progress athletically. Apparently, her strength and stamina weren't up to snuff for competitive tennis. The rumors are that Kaylie was pretty broken up about it and began searching for unconventional ways to correct the girl's athletic shortcomings. Which is when she came across IPE."

"And how did she learn about this, uh, clandestine institute?"

"That's one piece of the puzzle I couldn't get my hands on. What I can say is that her treatment supposedly involved promoting muscle growth by manipulating a gene."

Allisyn sat up straight. "That would be the gene controlling the production of myostatin, a protein which normally restrains the growth of muscles to prevent them from growing too large. The only example of it occurring in humans is a rare condition in which a spontaneous mutation of the gene leads to a myostatin deficiency and an overgrowth of muscle tissue."

"Would it be possible to somehow manipulate that specific gene in order to intentionally inhibit the production of myostatin and enhance muscle growth?"

"In theory, yes. But it's only been done in mice, and a good number of years ago, around 2004, I believe. Those animals were referred to as marathon mice because of the abnormal muscle growth, more colloquially known as 'Schwarzenegger' mice. Although its potential for treatment of muscle wasting diseases in humans has been proposed, no such studies have been performed so far."

"It is possible in humans, though, right?"

Allisyn stroked her chin. "I assume you're thinking about Felicity Edgers' tumor?"

"Mm-hmm. Apparently, the girl's strength and athleticism significantly improved after the treatment before her tumor was diagnosed."

"Ah, now I see where you're going with this. Malignant tumors are abnormal and uncontrolled growth of the original tissue, and rhabdomyosarcoma is a malignant tumor of the muscle tissue. I guess excessive stimulation of muscle growth through the genetic inhibition of myostatin could conceivably go awry and lead to development of such a tumor. I don't recall it happening with those mice, but it's an intriguing thought."

Martinez relaxed back in his chair. "Which brings me full circle to Amanda Leyfferts. Being such a visible public figure in her profession, she was really concerned with her looks, so much so she'd go to almost any extreme to prevent losing her youthful appearance. My sources say she was seeking a treatment to slow down, maybe even reverse, the aging process. I know you said this isn't always hereditary. But in her case, there's such a strong family history of it that I think it's fair to conclude her propensity for premature aging of her skin was genetic."

Allisyn understood his point and chose to elaborate. "And gene manipulation for the trait could have the same unintended consequence for her as it possibly did for Felicity. Overstimulation of skin cell growth in Leyfferts case, resulting in—"

"Development of abnormal skin cells such as basal cell carcinomas."

"Am I to assume your sources can confirm both Edgers and Leyfferts definitely had some sort of gene therapy at this IPE?"

"Uh-huh. And Apeloko as well."

"Kinda strange I've never heard of this place. I mean, I regularly review the genetic research literature and this place has never shown up. Although to be fair, I wasn't actually looking for it."

"Apparently, they've been pretty secretive in their operation and limiting their exposure."

"Then I guess your source is pretty good at what he or she does."

"Mm-mm," he smirked.

"Nevertheless, we'll need more concrete evidence of these treatments. And learn more about this IPE. May even need the help of your sources again."

"Not a problem. I'm already on it. . . . Are you saying you're with me on this?"

"Yeah, I guess so."

Martinez smiled and removed a pen and small notebook from his jacket pocket. "I'm going to jot down some to-dos for myself." He began writing. "Can you let me know if you find out anything more on your own about this IPE?"

No answer.

He looked up. "Dr. McLoren?"

Allisyn still didn't answer and instead just stared past him.

"Dr. McLoren? Are you okay?"

She looked at him, shaking her head. "I'm sorry. What did you say?"

"Can you let me know if you find out anything about this IPE place? . . . Is something wrong? You appeared distracted."

"Uh, no. I mean no, nothing's wrong. Yes, I'll check into it."

"It's a deal then."

They spent the next few minutes finalizing a plan to gather information and get back together.

As Allisyn walked the short distance home, her thoughts reverted to what distracted her before they parted . . .

CHAPTER

THIRTY-SEVEN

When Allisyn arrived at her office after her meeting with Phil Martinez, Ginger immediately approached her with a message from Constance Vasquez's assistant. The secretary wanted to see her first thing after she arrived.

"What's up, Ginger?"

"Don't know. It's all I was told. And to cancel all your commitments for the rest of the day, which I've already taken care of."

"Hmm. Guess I'll leave right now. Catch you later."

On the way over, Allisyn was trying to figure out what might be so urgent. She certainly wasn't looking forward to a repeat of their last meeting. No way did she want more pressure regarding the Nu-Genomix application. Whatever it was, she decided she would use the opportunity to share what she had learned about the company's research data cover-up. She initially intended to wait until she had the actual data in hand, but perhaps now was the time to let Vasquez in on the conspiracy.

"Secretary Vasquez will see you now."

Allisyn had been seated in the anteroom of Vasquez's office for barely five minutes when the receptionist beckoned her in. As she entered the office and the receptionist softly closed the door behind her, she was taken aback by what she saw.

As expected, Vasquez was sitting at her desk. But also present were Paul Westin and another gentleman she didn't recognize. Allisyn took a seat, totally bewildered.

"Good morning, Allisyn," said Vasquez. "I'm certain Dr. Westin needs no introduction. I've also asked Mr. Julian Shawe to join us. He's the CEO of Nu-Genomix, and I know you're familiar with his company."

Allisyn only nodded in their direction.

"You must be wondering about the nature and urgency of my request to meet, so I'll get right to the point. Dr. Westin and Mr. Shawe have come to me with some disturbing allegations."

Allisyn looked back and forth between Westin and Shawe, then toward Vasquez. "Allegations? Regarding what?"

"Not what, Allisyn. You."

"What are you talking about?"

"Did you recently have a conversation with Dr. Westin about the Nu-Genomix gene therapy application?"

"Yes. More than once."

"And what were the circumstances?"

"On the first occasion, Paul—Dr. Westin—called me to ask if I would participate with him at a conference to discuss gene therapy."

"And did you participate in the conference?"

"Yes. But you must already know that, since I'm sure he told you."

"Was it then you spoke with him about their application?"

"No. We actually discussed it when he first called me about the conference. After I agreed to participate, he inquired about the progress of the application."

"You didn't bring up the subject?"

"No. Why would I?"

Vasquez ignored the question. "Dr. Westin indicated it was you who initiated the discussion about the application during the call."

"What?" She glanced at Westin, but he was looking at Vasquez as if waiting for her to continue speaking.

"And as part of your conversation," said Vasquez, "you made the unsolicited offer to expedite review of their application and ensure quick approval."

Allisyn looked at Westin again, but this time he stared back at her. She turned to Vasquez. "What are you talking about? Why would I even consider something so blatantly inappropriate?" She raised her voice. "It was the other way around. He tried to convince me to intervene to expedite the review and approval."

"I see," said Vasquez. She looked over at Westin, but he spoke before she could ask him anything.

"Come on, Allisyn. You brought it up, offering to guarantee approval in return for a financial stake in the company's profits our gene therapy would ultimately generate. Don't deny it."

She moved forward in her chair, almost falling off the edge and looked at Vasquez. "You can't possibly believe what he said." She felt her face and neck warming. "It's an outright lie." She vigorously pointed at Westin, fully extending her arm. "He brought up the subject of my facilitating the application's approval, not me. And there was never a discussion of any remuneration. None at all."

Vasquez didn't say a word.

"You know that's not what happened, Allisyn," said Westin calmly. "It was your idea, and you were pretty upset when I insisted neither Nu-Genomix nor I would be a party to such collusion."

"Collusion? Why are you doing this, Paul? Who put you up to this lie?"

"I'm sorry, but you even emailed me afterward to follow up on your offer to guarantee approval of the application in return for shares in the company. Of course, I didn't respond. Nu-Genomix leadership would never even consider participation in such an arrangement. And I must admit I was shocked and personally disappointed, Allisyn. I never expected you of all people would present such a proposal."

"This is absurd." Her face reddening, she looked back at Vasquez. "Go ahead and check my emails if you want. You won't find any such communication."

Westin leaned back in his chair and crossed his legs. "They're from your personal email account, and we have copies."

"You must be kidding. This is crazy, completely bogus." She looked at Westin with disgust. "And did you also tell the secretary about the other conversation we had concerning your application? You know, how it was falsified by omitting certain damaging data and withholding it from the review team?"

Vasquez had been listening to this exchange dispassionately, but now jerked her head back and looked at Allisyn. "Falsified data? Could you elaborate?"

"Their application excluded data showing serious complications of their gene therapy in both animal and human trials, in some cases with fatal outcomes."

"Such an action is indeed concerning, Dr. Westin," said Vasquez as she looked back over at him. "It would be an egregious omission of important data at a minimum. Certainly a major violation of FDA protocol and regulations, I would imagine. Could you please explain?"

Westin remained amazingly calm. "I'm not sure what she's referring to, Madam Secretary. We didn't withhold any data, nor would we ever contemplate such deception. Our application was complete, and our commitment to the highest standard of data integrity and safety is unwavering. If something is bogus, it's her story. We never discussed anything of the sort."

Vasquez turned to Allisyn. "Do you have evidence of this missing data?"

Allisyn hesitated briefly. "No, but it was brought to our attention by an employee of the company."

"And you weren't going to take such information directly to the review committee?" challenged the secretary. "Why would you not disclose such critical information until just now?"

Shawe and Westin were staring at Allisyn, waiting for her answer.

Her voice faltered. "Because . . . I don't have hard evidence of the data in question."

"Can we get this individual, this employee, on the phone to corroborate your claim? Right now?" said Vasquez.

"No. It's not possible."

"Why not?"

"Because he's dead."

"Dead? My goodness. What happened?"

"Supposedly a biking accident."

"Hmm. Most unfortunate."

Westin crossed his arms, eyes intensely focused on Allisyn. "You're actually expecting the secretary to believe you accepted this information from an employee on hearsay alone? Hearsay from someone who's no longer alive to confirm the actual existence of such information?"

Allisyn turned away from Westin and addressed Vasquez. "It's complicated. Besides, I confronted Paul about this and gave him the chance to voluntarily withdraw their application until his team could sort out the problem."

Westin shook his head, smirking.

"And you made such an offer," said Vasquez, "because of your prior collaboration with Dr. Westin? Isn't that a bit of a conflict of interest? After all, if you truly knew there was a problem, I would expect you to go directly to the review team leader. Circumventing the proper course of action and instead inserting yourself into the process by addressing it with Dr. Westin, a former research colleague, seems to be a blatant disregard for the agency's own policy."

Allisyn ignored the comment suggesting her impropriety. "Gardener, the laboratory manager who apprised us of the data, had a hard copy of the files. As I said, he died before he could get them to us."

For the first time, Shawe spoke. "Bryce Gardener? A most unfortunate individual. We've been concerned about him for some time now. He was distraught over a recent divorce and had been acting rather strangely at work. We were preparing to arrange for him to have counseling and emotional support while he took some time off. Regrettably, not soon enough. I'm afraid the authorities suspect he may have taken his own life. . . . Without any hard evidence, this alleged bad data must have simply been a figment of his imagination given his disturbed state of mind. Poor man."

Allisyn sat motionless, her throat tightening.

"As for Dr. McLoren," continued Shawe, "perhaps she simply resented Dr. Westin, her former research colleague, for his success in the private sector and in developing this innovative treatment.

"Then she decided to guarantee our therapy would be approved in exchange for a financial interest in what she anticipated would be a successful, not to mention lucrative, venture. Of course, as Dr. Westin pointed out, we would never even consider participating in such an unscrupulous arrangement. Feeling twice scorned, once by Dr. Westin's success and then by our rejection of her proposal, Dr. McLoren must have been all too willing to accept Mr. Gardener's unverified story of such phantom data, sight unseen. And then she chose to use it as retribution toward Dr. Westin and Nu-Genomix. Of course, without actual proof of the data's existence, her ploy doesn't seem to ring true."

Allisyn was furious and nearly paralyzed by the absurdity of this entire scenario. "This is totally ridiculous! It's a complete fabrication to cover up the fraud they've committed by withholding damaging data which would discredit their work. I have a witness who spoke with Gardener and will corroborate all of this."

"Without hard evidence," said Westin, "I'm afraid such a witness would only be one more unwitting recipient of hearsay and Mr. Gardener's fantasized claim, a consequence of his unstable emotional state."

Vasquez listened intently to this exchange as she stroked her chin, then spoke. "Interesting theory, Mr. Shawe. But I must point out it's only a theory at this point. Of course, all possibilities will be considered as we look into this further. Thank you for agreeing to come here today. You may both leave now, and I will definitely contact you if further information is required."

Westin and Shawe thanked Vasquez for her time and left.

Allisyn leaned forward. "Constance, you can't possibly believe any of what they said. It's the most ridiculous story."

"I'm terribly sorry for all this, Allisyn. I truly am. Certainly you must understand their allegations are indeed serious, and I'm obligated to ensure they are carefully evaluated. Rest assured it will be a fair inquiry."

"And what about their falsified data? It would explain their motive for concocting this outrageous fabrication in the first place. To totally discredit me and divert attention away from their cover-up of the fraudulent application."

"Perhaps. But without proof of this data, I don't know what to say. . . . Unfortunately, there is one additional and rather serious issue to be addressed. If my inquiry corroborates what I heard from Dr. Westin and Mr. Shawe, it would seem you may not have been truthful when you testified to Congress."

"What are you talking about?"

"When you were responding to one of the senator's question about bias in the agency, you reassured the committee members you held no financial interest in any gene therapy product, nor would you consider doing so."

"Yes. I did. And still do. What are you implying?"

"Think about it, Allisyn. Your intent to trade approval of the Nu-Genomix gene therapy for such remuneration contradicts your statement to Congress. . . . If their allegation is corroborated, of course."

"You can't be serious." Allisyn scowled and started to stand up, then sat back down. "This is absurd. Of course I was truthful. Because their story about my soliciting financial compensation in return for approval of their application isn't true in the first place."

"I totally understand your indignation and anger at these allegations, Allisyn. And I'm not making any judgment at this time. Nevertheless, until there is something to definitively disprove what they're alleging, I have no choice but to initiate a thorough investigation. In the meantime, because we all know these kinds of issues can leak and adversely affect staff, I think it would be best if you take administrative leave from the agency."

Allisyn frowned. "Time off? For how long?"

"Until further notice. At least until we get all this resolved. We can't have any appearance of impropriety within the agency while we vet this entire situation. If it leaked out and became public knowledge you continued in your position under the pall of these accusations, it would be disastrous for the agency. The official story will be you're taking a planned personal leave of absence, with no mention of administrative leave or the accusations while it's being investigated. I certainly hope you understand. It's best if you recuse yourself for now, at least until this is resolved in your favor. Until then, it's important you have no contact with anyone at the FDA or involvement in its activities during your absence. And this matter should be kept confidential, of course, until we can substantiate what has occurred."

"But—"

"Unfortunately, Allisyn, I'm obligated to maintain the integrity of the agency until all of this can be cleared up one way or the other. I have no choice, at least until I hear anything to convince me otherwise. I hope you understand. My assistant will call security to escort you out. Unfortunately, policy dictates you're required to temporarily relinquish your pass cards under these circumstances. And your official email account will be temporarily suspended."

Without another word, Allisyn stood and walked out, wondering what bus just ran over her . . . and who was driving it.

CHAPTER

THIRTY-EIGHT

After she left Vasquez's office, Allisyn went directly home to her condo, calling Ginger en route. She didn't go into detail about the fraudulent data issue and the specifics of her suspension. Instead, she explained some personal issues had arisen requiring her to take a leave of absence. She would update her later. Allisyn figured it would be best to keep the details to herself for now. Ginger was understandably concerned and told Allisyn she would keep her advised of anything she heard around the office.

When she got to her apartment, she showered and threw on sweatpants and a tee shirt.

She padded barefoot to the kitchen, made herself some tea, and sat looking out her living room window. She was trying to make sense of the day's events and, more importantly, what to do next.

I need to enlist someone to help me deal with this. But who?

She reflected on her prior interactions with Vasquez, Westin and Krewe, all intended to pressure her into facilitating approval of the Nu-Genomix gene therapy. *But how were they connected?* Try as she might, she couldn't conceive of any shared motive.

Then she recalled her discussion with Senator Gradison about his chief of staff's attempt to coerce her. With all that transpired with Conyers, the missing data, and now Martinez with his IPE story, she overlooked the fact that Gradison never got back to her after their conversation. Although she figured it didn't matter much now that Krewe was dead. *I wonder if his attempt to coerce me and his death were related? And what about Vasquez? Did he ever talk to her?*

She decided to call him and see if he could shed any light on what just took place in Vasquez's office. When she did, Gradison was in a meeting and called back about forty-five minutes later.

"Thanks for returning my call, Senator," said Allisyn. "I'm following up on our conversation about the pressure I received to approve the Nu-Genomix application. Any updates?"

"I apologize for not getting back to you," he said. "It's been pretty hectic since Seth's death."

"What happened?"

"Apparently, he was being blackmailed with some past campaign finance issues to approach you. The FBI thinks he may have been despondent over that and committed suicide."

"Sorry to hear that. What about Secretary Vasquez? Do you have any better idea what her motive is?"

"Right. As I said, it's been pretty crazy around here and, well, I have to admit I never got around to speaking with her."

"I see." Allisyn wasn't happy but refrained from saying anything she'd regret. "Then let me tell you about my most recent experience with her." She proceeded to share what transpired in Vasquez's office with Shawe and Westin. He was quiet throughout.

"Hmm" was his only response when she finished.

"What do you think about this, Senator?"

He hesitated as if unsure about how to respond. "Well, this must simply be an unfortunate misunderstanding, Doctor. I can't think of any reason for her pressuring you as she did. And as far as your suspension . . . that's very unfortunate, but not to worry. I'm sure it will all be cleared up in no time. Let me talk with her, okay?

"Yeah, sure. Thanks. I'll wait to hear back from you."

Allisyn clicked off and tossed her phone onto the table next to her chair. *The most blasé response ever. Can't wait to hear what Vasquez tells him.*

CHAPTER

THIRTY-NINE

Allisyn was sitting at her kitchen table with a morning cup of coffee, thinking of her conversation with Gradison the day before. His response to her suspension was odd, to say the least. She felt put off at the time, and still did since she hadn't yet heard back about what he learned from speaking with Vasquez. Then she had an idea and grabbed her phone.

"Hey, Doc," answered Martinez after two rings. The reporter sounded like he was in good spirits. "Funny you should call. I was actually going to reach out to you a little later. I have some very interesting information to speak with you about."

"Speak" with me about? She wondered if news of her suspension leaked out and he heard about it. *Hopefully not.* Besides, she had something else on her mind.

"It's about IPE," he said, "and it's definitely interesting. . . . But what did you call for?"

Allisyn mentally breathed a sigh of relief. She was in no mood to tell him what had transpired with Vasquez quite yet. "I wanted to see if your sources could get some information for me. They seem to be pretty reliable."

"Indeed they are. What kind of information?"

"Let me hear what you have on IPE first."

"It's kinda detailed, actually. Best if we could meet to discuss it. Maybe catch dinner? There's this new place along the canal in Georgetown getting rave reviews, The District Bistro. You know it?"

"Uh-uh. But I'm game."

"How about this evening? Say sixish?"

"Have to check my calendar, but I have a funny feeling it's wide open."

He laughed. "Six it is. What's this information you're interested in?"

"I'll tell you later when we meet."

"A little mysterious today, are we?"

"Go on. I'll tell you about it tonight."

———

Allisyn left her car in a parking garage at the bottom of Wisconsin Avenue in Georgetown, just before the footpath along the canal.

The C&O Canal, now designated a National Historic Park, dates back to the mid 1800's. The narrow walkway along the Potomac river on the Georgetown side is regularly frequented by visitors out for a jog or a casual stroll. A good number of establishments on M Street above—eateries, bars and retail shops—have a back entrance along the walkway. Such was the case for the District Bistro.

She entered the restaurant ten minutes early after a short walk. Martinez had already arrived and was speaking with the hostess.

"Oh, hey there, Doc," he said, turning his head when she tapped him on the shoulder. His eyes travelled quickly up and down. "Hmm. Lookin' good."

"Seriously?"

He chuckled. "Appears we have a little problem here. They're running behind with their reservations, and it seems we'll have a thirty-minute wait."

Allisyn shrugged. "No problem. It's a nice evening. We can take a little walk until they're ready."

"Good idea. I like your 'so what' approach to adversity."

She responded with a slight smile. *If he only knew.*

After he gave the hostess his cell number, they left the restaurant and sauntered along the promenade.

Allisyn stopped and turned toward him. "Okay, let's get something straight between us right now."

His face slackened and he didn't say a word.

"Since we seem to have forged a working collaboration, from now on it's Allisyn . . . and Phil. You good?"

He shook his head and laughed. "You had me worried there for a minute. Sure, that's perfect."

"Okay, then." They resumed their walk. "Now tell me about IPE, Phil."

"Right. IPE is located a short distance outside Kuala Lumpur, the capital of Malaysia. For background, Malaysia touts itself as ranking among the best providers of health care in all of Southeast Asia. And medical tourism is a growing business for the country. It's been twice awarded the number one spot as Health and Medical Tourism Destination of the Year by the International Medical Travel Journal."

"Well, I'm definitely well acquainted with medical tourism, but I wasn't aware there was a trade journal dedicated to the practice."

"News to me, too. The country even has its own agency dedicated to *medical tourism.* The Malaysian Healthcare Travel Council or MHTC. According to their stats, Malaysia has grown its foreign patient volume each year since 2011. The council also endorses the facilities dealing in medical tourism in their country. They've doubled in the last few years."

"Interesting. I would have thought places like the Caribbean or maybe Central America would be more popular."

"Maybe. If you're looking for a nice vacation. But the number one driver of medical tourism in this day and age is cost. It's estimated health travelers who visit Malaysia save sixty-five to eighty percent on the same care compared to the cost in this country. They treat patients from all over, not just Indonesia. Including Europe and the U.S."

"No surprise," she said. "Technology has become much more affordable for other countries, although there's one exception to the pattern of less expensive care."

"What's that?"

"New treatments not yet approved in this country are being offered elsewhere without the regulatory oversight seen with the FDA. Take stem cell therapy, for example. It hasn't been approved yet for certain conditions here in the States. So individuals may choose to seek treatment outside our country despite the expense. In which case, it's called circumvention tourism. Of course, the inherent problem with such a scenario is the oftentimes unproven or even untested nature of the treatments being offered."

Martinez's eyes widened. "Which brings me to what my sources learned about the Institute for Personal Enhancement. But first," he said, stopping and looking at his watch. "I think we should start back. Don't want to lose our table."

"Apparently," he said as they walked back at a brisker pace, "it's not the typical medical facility offering care at reduced prices. Their treatments are high-end, financially speaking. More like a luxury spa offering all sorts of rejuvenative and self-improvement programs ranging from dietary and vitamin treatments to skin care and other body treatments. And various surgical treatments to boot, including cosmetic and weight loss procedures, among others."

As they reached the restaurant his phone dinged, and he looked at the text message, then said, "Table's ready. Let's continue inside."

After they were seated and had ordered, Martinez resumed his narrative as they each sipped a glass of wine.

"As I was saying, they perform a number of pricey surgical procedures. And here's the kicker. They offer a number of selective enhancement procedures using gene therapy."

"Gene therapy? Curious. As I mentioned when we spoke before, human genetic enhancement hasn't been universally accepted by the scientific community."

"Mm-hmm. Apparently, the MHTC was concerned about the exact same issue. It refused to endorse or even certify some of IPE's more questionable treatments. They were deemed not to have adequate scientific support and therefore refused to grant it a license to operate in the country."

"Then how did it end up there?"

"You're gonna love this. IPE is a Chinese operation and—"

"Chinese? If this MHTC was pushing back on China for its questionable regulatory oversight, why not just set up tent in China?"

"Probably because visas and travel are much easier for Malaysia, and ease of attracting international health care tourists to IPE was a key objective. As it turns out, China owns a significant portion of Malaysia's debt and—"

"Wait. Let me guess. They threatened to call in their debt unless they were approved to operate in the country."

"Mm-hmm. Very astute, Doc . . . uh, Allisyn. It would have crippled Malaysia financially."

She gently chewed on the inside of her cheek as she thought about what he had just said. "Makes sense. Without the kind of oversight our FDA provides, Chinese scientists have been much more aggressive in clinically applying genetic manipulation for various disorders. In fact, one of their scientists has even performed gene editing in embryos before birth. He tried to justify the procedure by saying it was to prevent HIV infection, but it didn't fly. There was an international outcry over the concern about unknown side effects and passing on changes to future generations. The negative reaction was immense, and the government was forced to put a halt to the practice. And now they're performing discretionary, non-medical genetic engineering? Pretty bold, I would say, considering there's currently an international ban on gene editing for elective human enhancement."

Martinez leaned forward. "My reporter instincts tell me there's a story here, a big story. I was thinking of taking a trip to see this place firsthand and wondered if you'd like to join me. I could use your medical and genomics expertise to get more information than I would. What do you say? Can you get a little time off away from work?"

"Oh, I think I can manage a few days." *More easily than you can imagine.* "However, I do have a request."

"Hmm. I'm listening."

"It's the information I was hoping you could help me with. I was wondering if you could use your sources to get it for me."

"About what?"

"Not what. Whom." She slid a folded piece of paper over to him.

He unfolded the paper and looked up after he finished reading it. "Interesting. How much do you want to know?"

"Everything."

He nodded. "How quickly?"

"As soon as possible. It's time critical and needs to be strictly confidential."

"Of course. Discretion is my middle name."

"Really? Mr. People in the News?" She grinned at him.

He ignored her comment. "I'm on it."

When they left the restaurant, neither noticed the man outside with a crew cut and turned up collar.

CHAPTER

FORTY

Kuala Lumpur International Airport in Malaysia is reached from Washington by way of a daunting twenty-two-hour flight, including one stop at Dubai International Airport. Martinez had prearranged a meeting with the Institute's medical director. During the long flight, they strategized their approach to learning as much as they could about the IPE operation. They decided he would focus on the public relations side and she on the medical details, especially their genetic enhancement procedures. As anticipated, they were both exhausted when they arrived, and went directly to the airport hotel where two rooms had been booked for them. The plan was to crash and get some rest, then visit IPE the following day.

After breakfast the next morning, they were met in the hotel lobby by the driver they had prearranged. IPE was about a thirty-minute drive from the hotel.

When they reached the institute, they were both impressed by the size and opulence of the grounds and facility. The main structure was surrounded by an extensive array of vegetation and planted gardens with fountains. The structure's lobby itself stood nearly three stories high, lined by glass with shining metal framing. The feeling was more like an upscale spa than a medical clinic.

They introduced themselves to the lobby receptionist, who confirmed their expected visit and led them to the office suite of the institute's director.

They weren't waiting long when a distinguished gentleman in a crisp black suit joined them. Allisyn suspected he was their host. "Good day," said the man. "My name is Rajaka binti Othman. I am the Operational Director here at the Institute." Although he spoke with a distinct accent, his English was more than acceptable. "And if I may ask, you are . . ."

"Martinez, Phil Martinez."

Binti Othman bowed gently in his direction. Then turning to Allisyn, he said, "Ah, you must be Dr. McLoren." He made a similar gesture toward her. "Your esteemed reputation in the field of genomics precedes you. Please accompany me to my office."

Once seated, binti Othman spoke. "I understand you want to learn more about our institute. What would you like to discuss?"

Martinez glanced over at Allisyn then back at him. "As I mentioned when I made arrangements for this visit, we anticipated meeting with your medical director."

"Ah, yes. Dr. Jaya Awang. Unfortunately, Dr. Awang will be busy performing procedures all day. But let me assure you I am prepared to answer any questions you may have regarding our facility."

"We appreciate it, Mr. binti Othman." He shrugged. "I'm writing an article for a prestigious American publication about medical tourism. My early research has revealed your institute to be the most frequent destination for those seeking medical care outside of their native country. We would like to learn about the services you offer."

Allisyn smiled politely. *Prestigious publication? Seriously?*

Martinez briefly glanced at Allisyn. "Dr. McLoren graciously agreed to accompany me to explain any medical issues which, I must admit, may lie outside my knowledge base. Are you certain there isn't a medical staff member who could fill in for Dr. Awang?"

"I'm afraid not. Dr. Awang insists on handling all medical questions about our services himself. Unfortunately. I do not have control over his schedule. However, I will do my best to accommodate your inquiries."

"Okay then," said Martinez. "Can you give us an overview of the institute?" He took out a small notebook and pen.

Binti Othman nodded. "As our name implies, our focus here is on individuals seeking a path to self-improvement. It can be intellectual, emotional, spiritual, or physical. Enhancement of oneself can have many facets, as you might well imagine. We like to think we offer a comprehensive array of options for our clients to choose from. Whether it be holistic methods such as yoga and meditation, medicinal and vitamin supplements, physical therapy and rehabilitation, or procedural interventions."

"Procedural interventions? Could you elaborate?" asked Allisyn.

"Surgical options, Doctor, such as . . . what do you Americans call it? Plastic surgery? I have always found the term 'plastic' an odd descriptor for a type of surgery. Here, we prefer the term 'enhancement surgery' in keeping with the goal of improving one's self image, sense of personal worth, or in some cases, physical performance."

Allisyn continued to probe. "I see. And what types of enhancement surgery do you offer?"

"Oh, we offer everything which is available in your country and much more."

"Much more? How so?"

"Because, and this is not meant to be an affront to you, Doctor, we are not hampered by what we perceive to be your unnecessarily restrictive American regulations. Many of our procedures have been developed and adequately tested, in our estimation, by our colleagues in China, with much fewer restrictions than would be the norm in your country."

Martinez jumped in. "Could we discuss the treatment several of your American clients—excuse me, patients—have received here?"

Binti Othman cleared his throat. "I am so sorry, but it will not be possible. We may not be equally restrictive in the procedures we perform as are your practitioners, but we certainly are not unscrupulous. We have our principles as well, and one is to protect the privacy of our clients. Similar to what you do with—what do you call it—HIPAA laws?"

Martinez smirked.

Their host tilted his head toward him. "Are you surprised I should know about your patient privacy laws, Mr. Martinez? You see, I spent some time in the U.S. learning about health care management before I assumed my position here."

Martinez uncrossed his legs and shifted in his chair. "Of course, Mr. binti Othman. I certainly understand." He looked over at Allisyn. "I believe Dr. McLoren has some more technical questions for you."

Allisyn obliged, taking a different approach. "Mr. binti Othman, thank you for the wonderful introduction to your services here at what appears to be an innovative institution of benefit to your clients. I understand you offer genetic enhancement therapy. Could you provide a little more detail?"

"It would be my pleasure, Doctor. Although far be it from me to explain what genetic enhancement is to you, of all people. I know gene therapy is a field of genomic science poised to offer hope to many individuals in your country suffering from diseases with a genetic component. We have added another dimension to such treatment—the use of genomic manipulation for non-disease purposes. Such as electively enhancing various traits, characteristics, and performance status indicators having a genetic component."

"I don't mean to challenge your practices, but how have you determined the efficacy and safety of such treatments?" She immediately thought this might be a bit too provocative. *Oh well. Too late.*

"I am aware the process of approval by your FDA is indeed deliberate and lengthy, Doctor. Our Chinese colleagues have a much more pragmatic approach, expediting the evaluation and approval process. And I venture to say we have benefited by our ability to now offer such genomic methods for the purpose of personal enhancement for those individuals who desire it." He paused. "I cannot be more specific, not only for the privacy of our patients, but also because of the proprietary nature of the treatments we utilize."

A bit of an evasive answer, but probably as good as we're going to get. "I appreciate your clarification." She looked over at Martinez. "Do you have any further questions, Phil?"

"Is it possible to tour the clinical areas of your facility?" he asked. "When I called to arrange this visit, I spoke with your assistant and understood a tour could be arranged. In all honesty, we very much anticipated the opportunity after having traveled such a distance."

Binti Othman frowned. "I'm afraid a tour would not be possible for the same proprietary reasons I mentioned earlier. Again, I am very sorry you were misled, Mr. Martinez. It certainly was not intentional. I will definitely speak with my assistant about not encouraging expectations we simply cannot meet. Perhaps I can provide you with our printed brochure we give to all individuals interested in procuring our services. It does an excellent job of describing our facility, resources, and available services. I believe it would be most helpful to you."

He reached over to his credenza and grasped two letter-sized envelopes with the institute's logo on the front and handed one to each of them. "This should be adequate for your purposes." He looked back and forth between his two visitors. "Do either of you have any further questions?"

Allisyn shook her head.

"Not at this time," said Martinez. "But if I do in the future, would you mind if I reach back out to you?"

"Not at all. Feel free to do so."

"Wonderful. And I'll be sure to provide you with my article when it's completed."

"Why thank you, Mr. Martinez. You are most kind. Now, if you don't mind, I have some affairs to attend to."

After exchanging farewells, Allisyn and Martinez left to meet their driver, who was waiting in the lobby to take them back to the airport for their flight home.

Binti Othman stood at a window overlooking the parking area, hands clasped behind his back. He was watching his visitors walk to their chauffeured car. His assistant was standing next to him. Without turning away from his view, he said, "Be sure I meet with Dr. Awang today as soon as he is available."

Then he placed a call to one of two men seated in a black sedan in the parking area below, exchanging very few words. Shortly afterward, the sedan left its spot, following Allisyn and Martinez's vehicle at a discreet distance.

Allisyn and Martinez went directly to the airport after they left IPE, even though they knew they'd have time to kill because their visit was much shorter than they had anticipated. When they finally boarded their flight home, she slumped dejectedly in her seat. "I guess this trip was a bit of a bust."

Martinez didn't respond immediately. He was looking down at his cell phone. "Maybe not." He put the phone in his pocket and looked up. "Just got an email from one of my sources. Says he's looking into something really interesting. But right now, I need to get some sleep." He closed his eyes and dozed off.

Allisyn tried but couldn't sleep. Her mind was racing, even though the thoughts seemed jumbled. There was a vague familiarity to what the IPE director told them, but her fatigue was getting in the way of making any connection. As she mentally reviewed his comments, it seemed she'd heard it all before.

Glancing over to Martinez who was sound asleep, she put on her earphones, tuned into the jazz channel, closed her eyes, and pulled the blanket up around herself.

CHAPTER

FORTY-ONE

By the time she returned to her condo in the afternoon after the long return flight from Malaysia, Allisyn was exhausted mentally and physically. When she awoke after sleeping for ten hours, she went for a much-needed run along M Street down to the waterfront, past Arena Stage and the District Wharf, then back. It was an early Spring day, perfect for the physical activity she sorely needed to clear her head. She showered and dressed when she returned, had a light breakfast, and sat down with a cup of coffee.

I need to tell him. She grabbed her phone.

"Uh, yeah?" said Martinez.

"Did I wake you, Phil? Come on! It's almost noon. I've already been out for a run."

She could hear him groan.

"You free today?"

"Uh-huh. Unless you count sleeping as being occupied."

"Funny. We need to talk."

"Okay, go ahead and talk."

"No. In person. We need to meet. How about lunch?"

"A late lunch."

Sounds like he's coming to life. "Old Ebbit Grille work for you?"

"Yeah, sure. Time?"

"Think you'll be awake and fully functional by, say, four?"

"It'll be close."

She chuckled. "See ya then."

The iconic Old Ebbitt Grill is the oldest bar and restaurant in D.C. It's located on the opposite side of the Treasury Building from the White House. Allisyn's fondness for the establishment dated back to her days as a medical student.

She was already seated when she spotted Martinez entering the restaurant. He was dressed in jeans and a light spring jacket over an unbuttoned teal polo shirt. He stopped just inside the door and scanned the tables.

Allisyn had to admit she found Martinez quite attractive when they originally met. But for the first time since then, she looked at him as more than just a reporter who had contacted her from out of the blue. Now she felt that vaguely familiar stirring inside that had been missing for too long.

She raised her arm and waved, catching his eye. He nodded and walked over.

"Why do you have to look so damn spry?" he said with an air of mock ridicule. "As if you got a good night's sleep."

"I did."

He grinned and they each ordered a beer.

Allisyn sipped her drink and looked down. He waited, but when she said nothing, he broke the uncomfortable silence. "You said you had something you wanted to share with me. In person."

She looked up. "Let's eat first." They both ordered steaks.

When they finished, Allisyn suggested they walk and she'd tell him her story.

Leaving the restaurant, they walked down Pennsylvania Avenue in the direction of the National Mall.

When they passed the Capital One Arena, Martinez raised his chin and tilted his head in its direction. "Ever been to a hockey game?"

"Yeah, kinda." She twisted her lips in a wry smile.

"Kinda? What do you mean?"

She laughed. "I played in college."

He abruptly stopped and turned to face her. "Are you kidding?"

"Uh-uh. Defense."

He shook his head. "Huh. Who would've guessed it? Defense, I mean. Center would seem more like it. We should catch a Caps game."

"I'm in. Had season tickets out in LA, but I've really been too busy here. Let's do it sometime."

"You bet. I can easily score some primo seats."

Allisyn went quiet, her demeanor suddenly very serious. "I'm currently on leave from the FDA, Phil. Indefinite suspension, to be more precise."

He stopped and turned to face her. "What? When?"

"Just before we went to visit the IPE."

"Why didn't you say something sooner?"

"I dunno. Guess I was still processing it myself. Didn't want to talk about it."

"What the hell happened?"

They reached the National Mall and Allisyn stopped them at 4th Street.

"Want a cup of coffee?" she asked.

"Uh, sure." Appearing confused, Martinez started looking around.

"How about my place? I make a mean cappuccino."

He tilted his head, eyebrows raised.

"Is that a yes?" she asked.

"I guess. Why not?"

"It's not too far a walk and—"

"I'm not certain walking is a very good idea." He was looking up at the sky, which had suddenly darkened with clouds.

"Let's walk fast then."

She led the way down 4th Street in the direction of the Southwest Waterfront and continued her story.

"Do you know anything about Nu-Genomix?"

He hesitated. "Uh . . . not really."

She gave him a questioning glance before continuing. "It's a biotech firm specializing in genomic research and development. The company's founder and CEO is a guy named Julian Shawe. They currently have a new form of gene therapy under consideration by the FDA."

She described how she was pressured—almost threatened—by Vasquez, Krewe, and Westin to expedite approval of the Nu-Genomix FDA application, adding how Westin was a former research colleague and current research director for the firm.

"In the meantime," she continued, "an employee of the company has come forward with a claim of damaging research data the company had suppressed. Supposedly, it exposed a potential but serious complication of the treatment."

"Supposedly?" Martinez looked puzzled.

"Yeah. He died before he could get the actual data to me."

"Hmm. Sounds suspicious."

"Exactly."

"What would you do with the data if you had it?"

"Get it to the committee reviewing the application. If it confirmed his story, it almost certainly would prevent approval of the application."

She explained how she confronted Westin, hoping to convince him to voluntarily withdraw the application. "Instead, he and Shawe went to Vasquez with a concocted story that I offered to approve their therapy in return for a financial stake in the company's profits."

"They claimed you were extorting them? And your boss actually bought such a ridiculous allegation?"

"Yes. Or at least gave it enough credibility to force an inquiry. And she rationalized my suspension by insisting it was necessary to mitigate any criticism of her leaving me active in my role if the accusations were ultimately proved to be true."

"How could they even prove it? It's their word against yours."

"Westin claimed to have emails I sent from my personal email account"

"Hmm. Must have hacked into your account and sent fake emails. Pretty serious stuff."

"It gets worse."

"Worse? Really? How could it?"

"After Shawe and Westin left her office, Vasquez suggested I had lied to Congress when I testified earlier in a Senate hearing and said I wouldn't have a financial interest in such a company while holding my current position."

"Lying to Congress? Is she serious?"

Allisyn shrugged and shook her head.

"So you need the actual data to expose their fraudulent application and debunk their story as just a ploy to get you out of the way. Right?"

"Yeah. Sure seems that's the case."

"Uh-oh," he said, holding his hand out. "Here it comes."

The sky had darkened even further and the rain came, slowly at first, but then in a downpour.

"We'll be drenched before we get there," she said. "Better hail a cab."

They got one pretty quickly, but not before they were soaked.

When they arrived at her condo building on M Street a couple of blocks north of the Waterfront, Allisyn convinced him to dry off in her condo while she made coffee.

Martinez was standing at the large window in the living room, staring out. "It's still really coming down."

She walked over to him with two glasses of wine. "Here."

"What happened to the cappuccino?" he asked as he turned toward her.

She grimaced. "Yeah, well didn't realize I was out of espresso, and you can't make cappuccino, at least good cappuccino, with American grounds."

He smiled at her. "This is fine."

There was a brief silence between them before she spoke. "Tell me about yourself, Phil." She sipped her wine. "Married? children?"

"Divorced. No children. Wife had a miscarriage. Our relationship went downhill afterward and fell apart."

"Oh, sorry. ... Guess I shouldn't have pried."

"Don't worry. It's been a while, and I'm over it."

"Any new prospects?

He took a sip of wine and looked up with a coy smile. "Possibly." . . . "And how about you? What's your story?"

Allisyn froze. *Trust. Can I trust myself?*

"Well? I'm waiting."

"Not married. I was engaged once, but it didn't work out." She paused, sipped her wine. "I was on a two-year research project in Rome and his job kept him in LA. Long distance separations will do a number on a relationship." *Yeah, and so will guilt.*

"Anybody now?"

She just shook her head.

Together, they gazed out the window at the reflected lights below, the only sounds the pattering of rain. And their breathing.

Allisyn suddenly became aware of her heart beating, quickening with each pulse. *Do I dare? Trust. Again.*

She turned toward him, took his glass and put it down with hers. She leaned in hesitantly and kissed him. Nothing more than a gentle brushing of their lips, then more firmly, and finally a shared, passionate, lingering kiss.

She pulled back and their eyes met for several moments, but neither spoke.

She took his hand and led him to her bedroom.

The sun was peeking through the curtains when Allisyn awoke the following morning. Martinez was still soundly asleep, lying on his side. She quietly got out of bed and walked over to her closet for a robe, not the least bit self-conscious about her nakedness. She looked back at him, but he still hadn't awoken. She softly padded out into the kitchen and put a pot of coffee on. As it brewed, she went over to the living room window and stood looking out. It had stopped raining and the sun was shining through the dispersing clouds.

A new day. Can it be? Her thoughts were once again interrupted by one word—*Trust.*

When the coffee pot beeped, she went over and poured two cups. She took them into the bedroom and set them on the bedside table.

The smell of strongly brewed coffee was pungent, and Martinez stirred.

She leaned over, lightly brushing his naked shoulder with her fingertips. He opened his eyes and looked up.

Her short robe fell open, diverting his gaze. He smiled.

"Last night was nice," she said, her voice barely above a whisper. "Very nice."

He looked back up, brushed a wisp of hair from her face, and gently pulled her onto the bed. "The coffee can wait."

Later in the morning, when she and Martinez were both showered and dressed, she made them a quick breakfast. They chatted about the IPE, but avoided discussing the night before.

As they were finishing up breakfast, her cell rang. The caller ID indicated it was Conyers.

"Doctor McLoren? This is Detective Hal Conyers."

"Yes," she mumbled through the small bite of toast she'd just taken.

"I'm checking in to see if there are any new developments at the FDA. I have some news myself. Are you free to meet?"

Am I free? Yeah, you might say that. "Actually, I'm available all day. Should I come down to Baltimore and meet you there?"

"If it works, fine. How about lunch on me at the Inner Harbor. You familiar with it?"

"Uh-huh. Been there several times. Love the Aquarium."

"Great. I'll meet you at the Harborplace entrance at noon. And I won't keep you too long so you can get back to work."

Back to work? Guess I'll have to tell him too. "Okay. See ya then."

When she told Martinez, they agreed to connect later in the day to discuss what the detective had to say.

He grabbed his jacket to leave, and at the door he gave Allisyn a gentle kiss. After he was gone, she leaned back against the door with a contented smile.

CHAPTER

FORTY-TWO

Allisyn was right on time for her meeting with Conyers, and he was waiting at the entrance to the Pavilion as promised.

"Good to see you again, Doctor," he said. "Let's grab a quick bite inside."

They each settled on a crab cake sandwich. When finished, they decided to enjoy the nice weather. They left the Pavilion and strolled in the direction of the Maryland Science Center, a wonderful collection of science-based exhibits and interactive learning opportunities.

"I've kept in touch with the FBI," said Conyers. "They're considering the deaths of Gardener and his sister suspicious, possibly homicides."

"Only suspicious? " she scoffed. "What else do they need? Written confessions? Of course they were murdered! To keep the fraudulent FDA application from being exposed."

"That's a solid working theory. But until we can prove what they're trying to cover up, it unfortunately remains just a theory. Gardener's death could, I say could, be considered accidental, and—"

"Seriously? Could?"

"I understand what you're saying, Doctor. However, without the actual data as evidence of a conspiracy to defraud the FDA, his death really could have been a simple bike accident unrelated to the Nu-Genomix situation."

"Uh-uh, no way. Sorry. I'm not convinced. . . . And Clarissa Brenner?"

"Well, her death is more definitively a homicide. Unfortunately, the perpetrator is unknown, so again, without the evidence to prove our theory, it can't be pinned on anybody at Nu-Genomix."

"In other words, you're saying what we already know. Without the hard data as evidence, we're at a standstill."

"Yes, and no. The FBI is still doing some background investigation. We'll see what turns up. But yeah, the data is key to sorting out those deaths."

"Why can't they just issue a subpoena for it?"

"My initial reaction too. Except it's not that simple. First, you'd need probable cause. Alone, the allegations of a dead man aren't enough. Besides, they could destroy the data as a preemptive maneuver. As Special Agent Parkes, the lead on their investigation, points out, right now the Nu-Genomix folks are probably assuming you don't actually have the data itself. Otherwise, you would have already come forward with it. And she thinks we shouldn't do anything to raise their suspicion to the contrary. At least until you can get your hands on it."

"Looks like we're stuck then."

"There is one other, uh, suspicious death you should know about. A lab worker at the Nu-Genomix facility in Teaneck, New Jersey. A guy named Aldo Peroni."

Allisyn frowned. "I didn't even know they had another lab. What's his connection?"

"Unknown at this point, although he may also have been working on their gene therapy project. The lab in Teaneck is the center of their animal studies."

"Then I gotta believe it's related. Gardener's notes indicated results of some of the animal studies had also been concealed. How did he die?"

"His autopsy revealed evidence of a massive heart attack, so we can't necessarily say it's suspicious at this point. Just have to keep it in mind until we learn more. But three deaths, all with a connection to this company? Can't be coincidence."

"You may have to add a fourth."

"What?" He stiffened and pulled his head back.

She told him how Seth Krewe had pressured her to ensure approval of the Nu-Genomix application, her subsequent meeting with Senator Gradison regarding Krewe being blackmailed and then Krewe's death. "FBI thinks it was a self-inflicted overdose. But I don't know. I'm skeptical. Too much of a coincidence."

Conyers had recovered from his surprise. "A little too convenient if you ask me."

"You're right there."

They turned left and continued walking past some boat slips.

"My turn," she said as they sat on a walkway bench with a view of the Aquarium across the harbor.

Allisyn described the pressure she had received from both Secretary Vasquez and Paul Westin, as well as Krewe. She finished by describing her confrontation with Westin about the missing data and the subsequent encounter with Vasquez when she was suspended in response to the fabricated accusation made by Shawe and Westin.

"Damn. How are you going to deal with it?"

"I'm not worried. Exposure of the fraudulent data will explain all of it."

As they left to walk back to their cars, Conyers said, "There really was a connection among the original three deaths I came across after all. Although I never imagined all this."

"To your credit, Hal, none of it would have come to light if it weren't for your persistence in pursuing it. Otherwise, we would never have known about the fraudulent data in the first place."

"I guess." He paused. "I've been wondering, though. Once you get this data as evidence, what happens next?"

"Well, first I would take it to the CBER Review Committee members. They review all the research data from a scientific perspective and determine whether or not to recommend approval of the therapy, clearing the way for it to be marketed for public use. They would then have to factor into their decision the nature of the data which was not originally disclosed and its impact on the actual merits of the product under review. Deferral pending further evaluation would normally be advised at a minimum. In this particular case, however, given the significant risk of patient harm, outright rejection is much more likely than deferral."

"Really? That's the only action taken after all this? Rejection of the application? Doesn't sound like much of a consequence for what's basically a conspiracy to commit fraud. Fraud is what we're talking about here, right?"

"No. I mean yes, it's a conspiracy to defraud the FDA. But no, of course it's not the only consequence. The fraudulent concealment and omission of relevant data in itself represents a criminal act."

"And?"

"The issue is referred to the FDA's Office of Regulatory Affairs and Compliance. According to its AIP, Application Integrity Policy, any data submitted with the intent to subvert the agency's review and approval of the premarket application is essentially considered a fraudulent act perpetrated against the government. Including any false research data or statement of material facts, as well as willfully omitting unfavorable test results adversely affecting the application. Which is exactly what has happened in this case. All such activities are data fraud and are designated as wrongful acts."

"What happens then?"

"The Agency's chief counsel would refer it to the FDA OCI, Office of Criminal Investigation. Working with the Justice Department, they would initiate a thorough investigation for evidence of the conspiracy. Not only are civil monetary penalties and other sanctions likely, but more importantly, criminal prosecution by the DOJ is highly probable. Not a good position for those at Nu-Genomix to find themselves in."

"Which explains their going to such extremes to prevent its exposure. Including getting you out of the picture."

"Yeah, it would seem that's the case."

"Then you really need to get your hands on a hard copy of the data to corroborate fraud."

"Mm-hmm. I just need to figure out how."

They were both silent for a moment.

"What about you?" asked Conyers. "Do you feel safe?"

"Right now, I figure they probably think I've been neutralized and no longer much of a threat to their plans, given I've been suspended and my credibility has been impugned, albeit falsely. And they're likely feeling pretty confident I don't have their data either."

"Maybe so, but it wouldn't hurt to get you a little protection."

"I'm good for now."

"Just let me know. No sense in taking any chances."

There was another brief silence. Allisyn nodded.

"We done then?" he asked.

"I believe so."

As they separated and walked in different directions, neither noticed they were being observed by a man with a crew cut and turned up collar.

CHAPTER

FORTY-THREE

The display read "Unknown Caller." Allisyn was sitting around at home thinking about her conversation with Hal Conyers when her cell phone buzzed. Thinking it was some form of spam call, her first instinct was to let it go. But in light of all that had transpired, her curiosity got the better of her and she went ahead and answered.

The caller's voice was oddly distorted, like an electronically altered computer voice used in movies. She could barely understand the speaker, and no way would she be able to identify the voice.

"Dr. McLoren," said the low-pitched, vibrating voice with a vague echo, "if you need further incentive to reverse your position on the Nu-Genomix application and agree to support its approval, please see the document delivered to your email once this call is ended. Make no mistake. Our resolve to use any means necessary to achieve that goal is firm."

The call ended abruptly with static. "Who is this?" she asked in a quavering voice. There was no response beyond continued static. When she scanned her phone's call log, the only identification of the brief call was the same as before—"Unknown Caller."

She immediately went to her laptop. With shaking hands, she logged in to her email account. She immediately noted a recently delivered message that had no sender identification. She opened the email, noting it had an attached document but was otherwise blank.

Under normal circumstances, Allisyn knew better than to indiscriminately open email attachments, but the ominous nature of the call and her current situation were too compelling to ignore.

When she finished reading the attachment, Allisyn slumped back in her chair, still shaking and now breathing heavily. It was an affidavit signed by a nurse alleging she had witnessed Megan on several occasions surreptitiously taking narcotics intended for patients from the medication station at the community hospital where she was assigned for an outside rotation.

Allisyn's initial shock was followed by a solid conviction this wasn't true. She wanted to believe it was simply a case of mistaken identity or misinterpretation of what Megan was accused of doing. In view of the mysterious phone message, however, she realized it was much worse.

This is clearly a ruse to intimidate me into reversing my stance on the Nu-Genomix application by threatening to use a bogus accusation against Megan. And that made this a very dangerous situation. First and foremost, she needed to protect Megan from this heinous accusation and expose it for the manipulated slander that she was certain it was.

She debated discussing it with Megan before acting but decided otherwise—at least for the time being—not wanting to upset or distract her. *No. I have to handle this myself.* And she knew her only recourse was to expose the Nu-Genomix fraudulent application, which would provide the motivation for this sham attempt to threaten Allisyn into inappropriately influencing the FDA's decision. Which took her right back to her original dilemma.

I need that damn data. Except now the stakes of this seemingly unachievable task had been raised and were more personal than ever.

CHAPTER

FORTY-FOUR

Allisyn was frustrated, angry, and frightened. Frustrated because she still hadn't heard back from Senator Gradison after he presumably spoke with Vasquez about her suspension. Angry at the threatening phone call she had received about Megan. And frightened at the prospect of what could happen to her niece if Allisyn failed to intervene and protect her.

Allisyn was underwhelmed by Gradison's response when she told him about her suspension. In any case, she concluded, he probably wasn't going to be helpful at this point anyway. Her attention reverted to the Nu-Genomix conspiracy and the missing data. As often happens when a specific problem is over-thought, however, she began second guessing everything she believed about the entire scenario.

Could Julian Shawe's story be true? Given his emotional state, could a distraught Gardener actually have dreamt up the existence of fraudulent data for some unknown reason? After all, so far, no one else had actually seen it but him.

Her train of thought was interrupted by recalling a famous quote from her favorite fictional character, Sir Arthur Conan Doyle's Sherlock Holmes. "There is nothing more deceptive than an obvious fact."

The absence of the damaging data from the flash drive left at Clarissa Brenner's murder scene is the obvious fact that supports Shawe's contrived scenario that Gardener fabricated the data. And per the fictitious investigators' dictum, clearly planted to throw me off the trail.

No way, she concluded. Shawe's proposition of Gardener fabricating the whole story was a non-starter as far as she was concerned. At least two people had died, four if Krewe and the Peroni fellow were included, presumably to prevent this data from getting to the FDA. And then there was Westin's outrageous reaction when she confronted him.

No. The data must be real, has to exist and I need to find it.

Without it, she had no credible way to substantiate the Nu-Genomix conspiracy and prevent approval of the flawed therapy. Not to mention exposing Shawe and Westin's ploy to get her out of the picture by trashing her reputation and career with their bogus story of her extorting them for a stake in the company. And probably most importantly, expose the false accusations against Megan as a way of getting Allisyn to move the application along to approval.

No matter how she looked at it, the data was key to proving the conspiracy and now crucial to proving the allegations against Megan were false.

There must be another copy.

As she thought about how she was going to get her hands on the data, something was nagging at her. She just couldn't put her finger on it, try as she might.

She went back to the beginning, her first meeting with Hal Conyers. As she replayed it in her mind, there was something there. But she couldn't get past the block in her mind's eye. Conyers said Gardener never gave him the data, just his handwritten notes. And something about how Gardener came across the data. As she thought it through, it seemed what she couldn't remember was related to how he found the data in the first place. But the more she tried, the more frustrated she got.

Then it clicked. Conyers mentioned Gardener found the data stored on a hidden drive housed within the company server.

No simple task if it was hidden, to say the least . . . Damn.
Why didn't I think of it when I met with Conyers earlier? She
immediately grabbed her phone and called the detective.

"I have a question I forgot to ask when we met. It's about
the data Gardener obtained. Didn't he tell you it was housed on
a hidden computer drive?"

"Uh-huh. Hidden and encrypted."

"And he had a friend help him locate the files, right?"

"Yeah. I think he said an IT consultant, and he, uh, hacked
their computer system and found it. The guy must be a real whiz.
He not only found the hidden drive but was able to break
through the encryption to get the data."

"That's what I thought you said. Did Gardener mention his
name?"

"Nah. At least not that I can remember."

"Sure?"

"I think so. . . . Wait. I recall something about him having
a background in military intelligence. I'm afraid nothing else specific, though. Sorry. What are you thinking?"

"I'll let you know after I figure it out. Thanks. Oh, and
thanks again for lunch."

Allisyn immediately did a web search for information technology consultants in the Raleigh-Durham area of North
Carolina. Since the region was rich in biotech and IT, she wasn't
surprised when her search produced fourteen separate hits. She
began the laborious task of calling each. Because Conyers hadn't
provided a name, the only inquiry she could make was if anyone
working at the company had military intelligence experience.

After twelve calls and two hours—much of it waiting on
hold—she came up empty. Of the remaining two, one was closed
for the day when she called. She was frustrated.

She called NB Technology Solutions, the last company on
her list, her fingers mentally crossed.

What sounded like a young woman answered. "Sorry, but I don't know if anyone here has been in the military," she said when Allisyn inquired. "It's kinda personal, you know? And unfortunately, I'm new here and the only one in the office at the moment. Can I have my boss call you when he gets back?"

"Sure," said Allisyn, exhausted and discouraged.

"Okay. I'll give him your number as soon as he gets in and make sure he calls you back today."

"Thanks." Allisyn flopped back in her chair and let out a big sigh.

Over an hour passed before her phone finally rang. "I understand you're inquiring about someone with IT and military intelligence experience," said the caller when Allisyn answered. "I was in the military, but I have to say it's an unusual request. May I ask what your need is for such expertise?"

"Let me explain. Do you know a Bryce Gardener?"

There was stone cold silence for what seemed like forever to Allisyn. "What about him?"

"My name is Dr. Allisyn McLoren, and I have reason to believe you may have assisted him in—"

"I'm afraid I can't help you. Good day—"

"No, wait. Please. Hear me out. I'm the FDA commissioner, and Mr. Gardener wanted to get some important information to our agency regarding an application from his company. He unfortunately died before he could accomplish that." She paused. "Before I go any further, let me say I'm very sorry for the loss of your friend. And if it's any consolation, there's suspicion his death was not accidental but intended to prevent him from providing us with the information. It's important the FDA gets it to avoid potential harm to many other individuals."

There was a short silence before he spoke. "How do I know you are who you say? And if his death wasn't accidental, that you're not part of it?"

"I totally understand, Mr. . . ."

"Burnes. Nate Burnes."

"Is Nate okay?"

"Sure."

"Here's what we can do, Nate, if it makes you more comfortable about my identity and reason for the request. Call the FDA directly and have them connect you to me. I'll call ahead to give them the okay. In the meantime, check my photo on the FDA website and we can do a video call to confirm I'm for real."

"Hmm. Okay by me."

Fifteen minutes after she made her call to the FDA operator, her phone rang with a video link. It was Burnes. "Well, does my picture do me justice?" she asked after she answered and could see him.

"Yes. Sorry to be difficult, but Bryce's death has had me pretty much on edge. I warned him something bad might happen if they found out, but he insisted on getting the information. Said it was really important to the application. Do you really think his death was intentional, possibly foul play?"

"The information Bryce was seeking had been excluded from the application submitted to the FDA, and he was correct about it being very important. I'm afraid it may have cost him his life. Unfortunately, he left a copy with his sister, Clarissa Brenner, and we believe she was also murdered to prevent us from getting it."

"What? That's terrible! What is this information, anyway?"

"Can't be specific, but it's some experimental data showing a potentially dangerous side effect of their treatment. If the FDA got its hands on it, approval of their application would be jeopardized and probably denied. Bryce uncovered the data and was trying to get it to us. The authorities, me included, believe both his death and that of his sister are directly related to the researchers' attempt to keep it from us."

"I see."

"Let me ask you something, Nate. Did you by any chance keep a copy of what you retrieved for him?"

Another brief silence. "Actually, yes. I thought it would be prudent if anything went sideways with whatever Bryce was planning. Little did I know . . ."

"Yeah. Always good to have a backup. If I arrange for you to meet me at the FDA to confirm everything we've discussed, including I am who I say, would you be willing to bring me a copy? And before you answer, let me say again that this was very important to your friend. He was trying to prevent a fraudulent application from being approved and causing harm to many people. I'll even cover your airfare."

"I guess. Under those conditions, I can do it."

"Thanks. Let's get it set up as soon as possible."

After they disconnected, Allisyn leaned her head back and sighed deeply. *Now I just have to figure out how to get myself into agency headquarters without being noticed.*

Shortly after Allisyn left Vasquez's office when she was suspended, she had called Ginger and given her the short version of what had transpired. She included the details of her meeting with Vasquez, Shawe, and Westin and their concocted rationale for her suspension.

They agreed the "official" word on her absence would be a temporary leave for personal reasons. At least until the whole situation could be resolved.

Now, since her suspension included no interaction with FDA staff, Allisyn's current plan required her assistant's help to get the flash drive from Burnes.

Ginger arranged to meet Allisyn at a service entrance to the building and covertly accompanied her to an unused conference room. Burnes was instructed to ask for Ginger when he arrived at the building lobby, who then escorted him to the same room where Allisyn was waiting, and left them alone together.

"It's a relief to meet you, Nate, although I'm sorry for the reason. The deaths of Bryce and his sister are terrible consequences of a conspiracy to defraud the FDA perpetrated by certain individuals within Nu-Genomix."

"I understand, Doctor."

"Can I take a look at the flash drive?"

He gave it to her and she popped it into a laptop she had brought with her. It only took a brief scan for her to realize it was the real thing. "This is it." She removed the drive and put it in her pocket. "I'll have to go through it in more detail, but this is what Bryce wanted me to have."

He nodded silently, a somber look on his face.

"I can't thank you enough, Nate. You've helped fulfill Bryce's mission, and it will make a huge difference to a lot of people. Let me reimburse you for your flight and—"

He gestured with his hand for her to stop. "No, but thanks anyway. This is the least I can do for Bryce. I hope you accomplish what you need here. Be careful and stay safe."

Allisyn called Ginger back to the room and asked her to escort him out.

"Finally," said Allisyn as she left.

When she returned to her condo, Allisyn immediately put the flash drive in her laptop. She methodically reviewed the voluminous amount of data present. When she compared it to Gardener's written summary, they correlated perfectly. "Yes!" she said loudly, accompanying it with a raised fist pump.

CHAPTER

FORTY-FIVE

After reviewing all the data on the flash drive, Allisyn collapsed onto her favorite lounge chair and stared out the large window across the room. She was now convinced she finally had the evidence needed to prove the Nu-Genomix fraudulent conspiracy. Equally important, it would substantiate her effort to have her suspension rescinded by Vasquez. Not to mention debunking the nurse's falsified statement about Megan.

Despite the urgency of these objectives, her thoughts kept returning to the question nagging at her since the flight home from Malaysia and their visit to the Institute for Personal Enhancement.

She took out the brochure the IPE director gave to her and Martinez and read it cover to cover. Most of it was typical marketing material. When she came to the section on genetic enhancement, it was very basic, describing the process in layman's terms and only in a general manner. No specifics, and the brochure referred the reader to an IPE provider for additional information.

And then it came to her. The conference panel with Paul Westin. Specifically, his tirade about the feasibility and practical application of non-therapeutic human genetic enhancement. *Almost like an advertisement for the institute. Coincidence?* She thought it was possible but needed to be sure there wasn't more to it than that simple explanation. And she had an idea how to find out.

After pouring a cup of coffee, she went back to the desk in her study and fired up her laptop again. This time she signed in to her FDA account, anxiously waiting to see if she was locked out because of her suspension. The sign-in was taking longer than usual and she started fearing the worst, when suddenly her home page popped up. Apparently, only her email account was locked. She breathed a sigh of relief, then logged on to PubMed, the interface used to access the National Library of Medicine's extensive MEDLINE database of scientific articles, references, and other biomedical content.

She did a search by author, typing in Paul Westin. Not surprisingly, the search took several minutes to complete, returning a voluminous number of articles, a number of which were co-written by her and related to the Nobel Award-winning research they had done together. She decided to narrow the search by typing in his name plus "human genetic enhancement" plus "human genetic engineering." This search was quicker and returned a lesser number of articles, mostly editorials and scientific opinion pieces on the topic. Nothing referenced original research on his part in this area of genomics. As she scrolled through the list, however, two results caught her attention. After reviewing both articles, she printed them out, put them in a folder, and decided to do one additional search.

She Googled IPE and found the website to be essentially a web version of their brochure. Although genetic personal enhancement was described as one of the procedures offered, as a source of information it was as basic as the print brochure. She dug deeper under the "About the Institute" tab, and after more searching and sifting through less meaningful information such as descriptions of the facility architecture and surrounding landscaping, found a page listing the management structure. The gentleman she and Martinez met with, Rajaka binti Othman, was listed as operational director, as he had presented himself. The same for Dr. Jaya Awang as medical director. She shook her head as she recalled how they were unfortunately not able to speak with him. She had hoped to query him on the scientific and medical details of their genetic enhancement procedures. *Oh well. Too bad.*

She continued scanning the IPE organizational structure, and her eyes widened when she came to a section labeled "Board of Directors." She considered it a lucky find because it was pretty well buried among the other extraneous information. Following the list of board members she noticed an additional section labeled "Other." After digesting what she read in both sections, she leaned back in her chair, took a deep breath, and sighed. She printed out both these sections of the organizational document and added them to the folder with the articles.

She immediately called Martinez. "Hey," he answered."

She didn't wait for him to say anything else. "I need you to get your sources working for me again."

"What do you need?"

"As much detail about IPE as possible, including financials, investors, stuff like that. The kind of business information you won't find on their website."

"A pretty tall order, Doc."

"You always tout the skills of your sources. Now prove it."

He chuckled just loud enough for her to hear. "Sure. I'll check into it pronto. By the way, I'm expecting that other information you requested any day now. Maybe I'll have both of them for you at the same time."

"Great. And I also have some updates that you're sure to find very interesting. Catch you later."

Sitting in a black sedan on the street below Allisyn's condo, an opened laptop equipped with digital network intrusion software positioned next to him on the passenger seat, Jason Tinley had been intently staring at a real-time screen capture of Allisyn's computer.

CHAPTER

FORTY-SIX

Satisfied she now had the hard evidence of the damaging research data Nu-Genomix had intentionally excluded from the FDA application, Allisyn's first order of business was to let Constance Vasquez know so she could have her suspension lifted.

She called and left a message with the secretary's assistant to return her call as soon as possible, stressing it was an urgent matter. As the day wore on, she heard nothing from Vasquez, so she called the assistant back to confirm the message had been passed on.

It was getting late in the day, and with still no call from Vasquez, Allisyn called again, but now got a recording the office was closed.

Damn. It's like she's avoiding me. She decided to text Vasquez directly. "Need to talk. It's urgent. Call me ASAP."

When she received no response, she sent another text.

"Urgent! I have the damn data now. Confirms Gardener's allegations it was intentionally withheld by Westin and his team. I want my suspension lifted immediately. Call now or I go public."

Is she crazy to ignore me? Or does she think I'm bluffing? She tried one last text.

"We can meet and I'll show you the data. It's real."

About two hours after she sent the last Vasquez text, Allisyn's phone rang. *Finally,* expecting Vasquez. She frowned when she saw the caller ID indicated it was Martinez.

"What the hell happened?" he asked.

She explained how she had obtained the data from Burnes and her attempts to reach Vasquez to get her to lift the suspension because the data would prove the conspiracy. And discredit Shawe and Westin's bogus claim she attempted to extort them.

"Yeah, well, it doesn't appear you got the reaction you hoped for. Vasquez just released a statement to the press for immediate publication announcing your suspension and spelling out the reason. Looks like your threat backfired."

"What?" Her back stiffened and she felt the warmth rising in her neck. "Why would she even consider doing that? The message I left said I had the data to prove the falsified Nu-Genomix application and disprove their sham story."

"Maybe she didn't get your message. Or she's calling your bluff, which is more likely. Either way, it's public and will be much more difficult to repudiate, even with the data, than if it hadn't been announced."

"Damn."

"Nothing you can do about it now." He paused. "Oh, by the way, I've got that information you asked for."

"All of it?"

"Unfortunately, only the first set you requested. Not the info on IPE, but it should be soon. I took a quick look, and I think you'll find it fascinating and extremely useful. I'll email it over to you shortly. Gotta go now. I have a few details I need to attend to. Let's get together first thing in the morning."

Allisyn kept checking her email, but nothing from Martinez until about thirty minutes after they talked. His email was accompanied by two files. Each consisted of three pages—a cover page and two pages of text. She printed both files and settled in to read them.

When she looked at the pages, she was confused. The cover page of one file said "Bartone." The second cover page said "Williams."

"What the hell?" she said aloud. "Who are these people? This isn't what I asked for."

She grabbed her phone and was about to call Martinez, figuring he sent the wrong files, when she quickly thumbed through the pages of each document and realized she didn't need to call him after all.

CHAPTER

FORTY-SEVEN

Lying in bed, eyes wide open and staring at the ceiling, Allisyn was exhausted. She still hadn't fully adjusted to the time differential after returning from Kuala Lumpur, and what she learned from the documents Martinez had sent over the night before didn't help her sleep either.

She dressed casually after taking a quick shower, then brewed some coffee. She began writing notes for Martinez summarizing what she had discovered with her earlier MEDLINE search when her phoned dinged, indicating a new text message. She opened it and almost dropped the phone. Attached was a photo of Megan, mouth covered with duct tape. She looked terrified.

The message was simple, and horrifying.

"If you want to see your niece again alive, come down to your car now."

Allisyn gasped and covered her mouth with her hand before reading the rest.

"If you communicate in any way with anyone, I will know and you will never see her again."

Her hand was shaking and her coffee spilled.

She immediately slipped into a pair of shoes and took the elevator down. As she approached her car in the parking garage, she noticed a man with a crew cut leaning against the closed driver's door, arms folded across his chest. Even in her panicked state, she noticed his shirt collar was oddly turned up.

When she reached the car, Tinley tapped on the back seat window, drawing Allisyn's attention. She immediately recognized Megan, mouth covered with tape and looking at her with wide, pleading eyes. She was banging on the window with her bound wrists.

Allisyn's knees went weak and she felt a knot in the pit of her stomach. She looked furiously at the man and demanded, "What do you want? Whatever it is, let her go and deal with me."

"Well, that is something to consider . . . but no. Get in the car. We're taking a little ride."

"No! Let her go first." She was visibly trembling now.

Tinley scowled and shook his head. "You know, Doctor, you had your chance to avoid such a messy situation. All you needed to do was make sure the Nu-Genomix application was approved. After all, you had enough, uh, encouragement. You even had a nice little vacation from work. And then there's your niece's little indiscretion. If you had cooperated, I suspect you'd be back at your job by now, business as usual. And she wouldn't have to worry about that nurse. Instead, you started sticking your nose into places you didn't belong, and got mixed up with a misguided reporter on top of everything else. So now I'm afraid we have to rectify the situation. Permanently."

As he finished, her eyes were drawn to the opening of the garage where a man with a gun was entering. *Oh my god! It's Detective Conyers.*

Unfortunately, Tinley noticed the direction of her eyes and followed them to Conyers. He unfolded his arms, revealing a revolver in his left hand. He quickly fired off a shot. Conyers dropped his gun and it bounced away. Grunting, he dropped to his knees, holding his right shoulder with his left hand, his right arm hanging limp as blood oozed out between his fingers. He rolled over on his side. He was breathing heavily, but didn't move.

Just then, another man stepped out of the shadows some distance away from where Conyers was lying. The garage's dim lighting precluded a clear view, but Allisyn could make out that he was also armed.

"FBI. Drop the gun, Tinley."

Staring at the man, Tinley turned his gun towards Allisyn and reached out to his side to pull her close.

Thinking quickly, she backed away, taking a short step to the side beyond his reach, causing him to turn and look at her. The savvy maneuver produced her intended result, momentarily diverting his attention from the agent. As he did, a shot rang out, hitting Tinley square in the chest. It all happened so quickly it was just a blur to Allisyn.

The impact spun Tinley around and threw him up against the car. The gun fell from his hand, he bounced off the car and collapsed in a heap. Blood was visible under his turned-up collar, and he wasn't moving.

The agent pulled out his phone and hit speed dial. "Suspect and officer down. Need assistance."

In a slight jog, he came over to Allisyn. "Are you okay?"

She blinked and quickly shook her head. "What the hell?"

"Let me check on your niece."

He opened the car door, let Megan out, and removed her gag and the zip ties binding her wrists. She immediately ran to Allisyn and they embraced. Megan was shaking terribly. They moved a few steps away as the agent came over to check the assailant.

Sirens could be heard in the background.

Allisyn separated from Megan and walked over to the agent after he finished checking Tinley for a pulse.

He stood and shook his head. "Nothing."

"FBI?" she said. "Seriously?"

The agent holstered his revolver. "Mm-hmm," said Martinez. "I'm afraid so. Been working undercover on this deal for the last year."

"What deal? And whatever it is, what do I have to do with it? And why did you get me involved in the first place?"

Just then, the police, additional agents, and an ambulance arrived.

"I'll tell you what," said Martinez. "Let us get this place cleared out. Then we can sit down and I'll explain it all. It's complicated."

CHAPTER

FORTY-EIGHT

It took nearly two hours to clean up the garage and for Martinez to debrief the support team. Conyers was taken to the nearest hospital. Other than the bullet wound to his shoulder, he would be fine. The EMTs had slowed the bleeding down with pressure, and their on-site evaluation determined the blood flow and nerve function in his arm were normal.

Martinez joined Megan and Allisyn at the kitchen table in her condo. They each had a steaming cup of fresh brewed coffee in front of them.

Megan was rubbing her wrists, which were slightly reddened where the zip ties had bound her hands together. Occasionally, she shuddered and wiped a tear from the corners of her eyes.

Allisyn sipped her coffee, then looked up at Martinez. "Well? Do you want to share with us what the hell is going on?"

Martinez took a deep breath. "I'm an FBI agent, and—"

"You've already told me that, dammit! What I want to know is why you deceived me into believing you were a reporter angling for a story on the institute in Malaysia all this time."

"I didn't mean to deceive you, Allisyn. I—"

"Then what the hell do you call it? A game of charades? A deadly game, as it turns out." *And you even slept with me. Trust. Again.*

"I'm sorry, Allisyn. The Bureau has been working with Interpol and the WHO for the last six months on what's going on at IPE. At first, only the WHO was involved. They were really concerned about the frequency and severity of complications showing up as a result of the genetic enhancement procedures being performed there. And as you and I have discussed, human genetic engineering hasn't been sanctioned by the WHO or any other international organization."

Allisyn's anger had subsided, her voice softened considerably. "Why didn't they just close the whole operation down?"

"It's not that easy. Some of the operation's other connections in addition to the Chinese were pretty heavy hitters— financially and politically— and were blocking investigations. That got Interpol to start looking into it."

"And where do I come in? Why did you get me involved?"

"That's where it gets a little complicated. Interpol's investigation revealed some IPE investors are here in the U.S., and reached out to us for assistance. When Detective Conyers came to us at the FBI following Clarissa Brenner's murder, he shared her brother's death as well and its relationship to the missing data and the Nu-Genomix conspiracy to defraud the FDA. It was a big red flag for us."

"You were at the same meeting? With Conyers?"

"Mm-hmm. Along with another agent and Deputy Special Agent Alondra Parkes."

"Did you tell Conyers about this IPE investigation?"

"No. Not exactly."

"What does that mean?"

"Well, I had a brief conversation with him after the meeting and explained how we were looking into another issue that could possibly be related to what he told us about Nu-Genomix. But I didn't provide any specifics. I did suggest we stay in touch with each other and share information as necessary."

She shook her head and rolled her eyes. "And you told him about working with me?"

"No, not then. I hadn't contacted you yet. Actually, we weren't convinced there was a connection until shortly after that meeting, when we shared what he told us about the Nu-Genomix data issue with the WHO. They felt the complication that was being withheld from the FDA had distinct similarities to what they saw coming out of IPE. Not too long afterward, Interpol asked us to work with them on the Nu-Genomix angle to see what we could come up with."

"And you decided to use me as a source of information on Nu-Genomix?"

"Well, the firm did have an application pending with the FDA for its new gene therapy, and you are the commissioner, with a genomics background and a work history with their research director. So yeah."

"Why didn't you just tell me about it?"

"Uh, that's not quite the way undercover works, I'm afraid."

"You're saying you couldn't trust me?"

"Come on, Allisyn. That's not what I meant. Trust has nothing to do with it. I just couldn't compromise the cover identity I had already established. It all went more smoothly if you believed I was who I was pretending to be. Besides, the last thing we wanted was for the bad guys to learn you were working with an FBI agent. I mean, a reporter was chancy enough."

Trust. Always my problem. She sighed. "What about today? How is it you and Conyers were both here?"

"Shortly after I first contacted you and we began, uh, collaborating, I let him know, and to keep it confidential. Right then we agreed you should have some protection."

"Protection? Like I'm a child?"

"Be real, Allisyn. Look at the deaths up to this point as a direct result of this conspiracy and cover-up. Even though you were suspended, I suspect they weren't convinced you would stop trying to get that evidence. It was inevitable they would want you out of the way permanently sooner or later. So Hal, another agent and I have been trading off protective surveillance on you."

"Hmm." She was shaking her head. "And Megan? She shouldn't have been involved in any of this." She traded glances with her niece.

"Actually," he said, "she's had coverage as well. It didn't take much to figure out they'd use her to get to you. Exactly what happened today. He grabbed her and we followed them here."

"And you weren't worried he'd harm her first?"

He looked at her niece. "No offense, Megan, but to them you were just a way of getting to Allisyn. Then he would deal with both of you together."

Allisyn hesitated briefly before telling them about the email she received threatening to have a nurse accuse Megan of stealing narcotics at the hospital if the Nu-Genomix application wasn't approved.

"What?" said Megan. "That's ridiculous. I never did any such thing."

"Don't you think I know that? Another reason I needed that data."

"Probably the same guy who grabbed you today," said Martinez. "He must have had something on the nurse and blackmailed her into making the false accusation to put more pressure on Allisyn."

"Who was he, anyway?" said Megan.

"A Nu-Genomix henchman. Went by the name of Tinley, Jason Tinley. Has a shaky military history and did mercenary work before settling in at Nu-Genomix. We believe he was involved in all the deaths. Gardener, Brenner, Peroni, Krewe."

"Krewe? I thought his death was a suicide."

"Apparently, Tinley was pretty talented along those lines. Making a murder appear to be suicide. Or murder look like a bike accident."

"Gardener?"

"Uh-huh. And Peroni, the lab tech in Teaneck. Made that look like the guy had a heart attack. Except the autopsy showed he had enough cardiac stimulants in his system to knock off a horse—figuratively speaking."

Head down, Allisyn rubbed her forehead. "You know that information I said you'd be interested in?"

"Yeah. I've been wondering about that."

"Well, I did a little investigative work of my own. Found two articles in the scientific literature authored by Paul Westin on the topic of human genetic enhancement. One was his keynote address at a major scientific symposium in Beijing, China, three years ago. It was entitled *Human Genetic Engineering: Is the Future Here Now?* The other was his script of a talk entitled *The Endless Potential of Human Genetic Enhancement.* It was presented to the board of directors of IPE. Both articles were incredibly supportive of the technology. In fact, the wording was almost identical to what he said at a panel discussion we recently participated in together at Georgetown. We had a pretty heated discussion on the pros and cons of elective human genetic engineering and enhancement. You can probably guess what side of that issue he landed on. Aggressively so, actually."

"Really? We didn't know about those articles."

"Like I said, I had to do a detailed literature search and know what to look for."

"Impressive."

"There's more."

"Hmm. I'm listening."

"I scoured the IPE website and discovered two other tidbits. Again, somewhat obscured. There was a document on the organizational structure of the institute with two sub-sections. The document itself was not prominent on the site and I was lucky to find it. The first section was labeled as board of directors. There were eleven names, ten of which were either Chinese or Malaysian. It was the eleventh name that immediately caught my eye—J. Shaw. At first I was skeptical of any connection since Julian Shawe spells his name with an 'e' at the end, and the initial "J" could certainly stand for any number of first names. But that would be too much of a coincidence, and I'd bet anything it is Julian Shawe."

He nodded. "Agreed. We'll get our Interpol connection to confirm. What was the other section?"

"It was literally labeled 'other,' and held several additional names, all with titles of no relevance I could imagine. Except for the last one—Scientific Adviser to the Board. The associated name was Paul Westin, PhD.

"Damn. And Interpol didn't catch that, either? Looks like we should sign you on as an investigative consultant. Become one of our sources."

Megan broke out of her sullen state and smiled.

"Yeah, right," said Allisyn. "And that's your connection. IPE is using the exact same gene therapy technique Nu-Genomix is trying to get approved here. Has to be, with Westin involved with them."

"Agreed. Sure looks like it."

"Except IPE hasn't had to deal with the same regulatory controls as with the FDA." She paused as if in thought. "Interesting. Leyfferts, the Edgers girl, and Apeloko. They all had complications explained by an off-target effect of their genetic enhancement procedures. Likely the same for all the IPE patients identified by the WHO as having similar complications. The same type of genetic misadventure that occurred in the Nu-Genomix trials. And the data they omitted from their application is the proof. Not only would it scuttle their FDA application if exposed, it would force the WHO to push for closing down IPE for using a non-sanctioned procedure known to be unsafe."

"Totally makes sense." said Martinez. "They needed to prevent you from getting your hands on the incriminating data at all costs."

"Yeah. Explains the bogus story Shawe and Westin concocted about my trying to bribe them into giving me a piece of the action. They must have figured Vasquez would be obligated to investigate their claim, and a suspension would get me out of the picture and discredit anything I said about their deception."

"And then they decided to add an extra incentive to prevent you from nixing their application by threatening to use that nurse's false accusation against Megan."

Allisyn looked over at her niece. "Sorry, Megs."

"Except," said Martinez, "somebody calling the shots at Nu-Genomix decided you still posed the risk of somehow finding out about the connection between them and IPE."

"You mean discrediting me with their fabricated story and removing me from the FDA wasn't enough?"

He shrugged. "Maybe they somehow found out what you discovered about Shawe, Westin, and the IPE board. Hell, I wouldn't be surprised if this Tinley fella has been watching your every move this whole time. If that was the case, they couldn't take the chance you'd use that information to expose the entire operation. My guess is it was decided a more permanent solution was necessary to eliminate that possibility." He looked over at Megan. "Unfortunately, they used your niece to get to you. In the end, the data was the key to all of it. With it, they knew you'd have proof of the fraudulent application and their conspiracy to cover it up. But once they knew we visited IPE, they probably figured you were dangerously close to discovering the connection between their gene therapy and IPE, which was the real profit engine of this entire scheme. And they were right."

Allisyn reached over to a nearby table and picked up the two documents Martinez had emailed over the night before, one labeled Bartone, the other Williams. She waved them at him. "And these? Are you kidding?"

"Not even a little bit."

She tossed them on the table, shaking her head.

He pulled an envelope from his pocket. "This is the intel on IPE I told you I had. It's pretty detailed, so I'll just summarize it."

"More? There's really more?"

"Oh, yeah. According to Interpol sources, there's another party besides the Chinese associated with IPE. A British organization called Future Care. Initially, it was thought to be some form of European investment group with ties to China."

"China has outside investors?"

"Actually, Interpol couldn't identify any."

"If not any investment vehicle, then what is this Future Care?"

"It's a part owner of IPE along with a Chinese organization and helps manage the joint venture. Turns out Future Care is a shell corporation for the actual co-owner . . . Nu-Genomix."

"Well that confirms everything we just discussed. IPE is using the Nu-Genomix gene therapy technology, flawed as it is, while Shawe and company share in the profits."

"Mm-hmm. And now you have the entire picture, all tied up in a neat little bundle."

"Except for these." She again held up and waved the two documents marked with names he emailed to her. "Appears I have some loose ends myself to take care of."

Megan had stopped rubbing her wrists and was listening attentively. "What happens now?"

"Deputy Special Agent Parkes will put all this together and get it to the WHO and Interpol, and they'll take whatever action they deem appropriate with IPE and China. As for Nu-Genomix, what do you think, Allisyn?"

"Well, since I now have the data, I can take it to the CBER Committee, and it will definitely stop the Nu-Genomix application in its tracks. No way they'll approve their gene therapy, knowing about the potential complications. As for the conspiracy to defraud the agency by withholding critical data, I'll turn it over to the agency's chief counsel, who'll work with the FDA's OCI—Office of Criminal Investigation—the FBI, and a Department of Justice prosecutor to bring action against all the pertinent parties at Nu-Genomix, from Shawe and Westin on down, for criminal conspiracy to defraud the government."

Martinez nodded. "And it most certainly will result in both criminal prosecutions and civil actions, including hefty fines on the company if it survives the scandal at all. Not to mention conspiracy to commit murder as part of another criminal act. Even though the murderer, Tinley, is dead."

Allisyn sighed heavily and looked at Megan. "How ya doin, Megs?"

"I'm fine now. I must be. My wrists don't hurt anymore, and I'm getting hungry."

They both laughed.

"Let me get you back to your apartment, and we can stop on the way for something to eat." She looked over at Martinez. "Will you join us?"

He grimaced. "As much as I'd like to, I'll have to take a rain check. I need to get back to the bureau to work on a report for what went down here. And I want to stop by the hospital to check on Hal."

"Right. Rain check accepted." Allisyn smiled at him. "Just let me know when."

CHAPTER

FORTY-NINE

Once Martinez left, Allisyn drove Megan back home. They stopped at a sandwich shop near the Georgetown campus for a bite to eat. Then she stayed with her niece for a while to make sure she was comfortable. Allisyn suspected her emotional state was still a little fragile from the harrowing experience she had gone through.

Martinez reassured them both Megan would continue to be under protective surveillance even though Tinley was dead, at least until the FBI and DOJ could move on Nu-Genomix. And they would get the nurse in to tell them how Tinley had coerced her to make a false statement about Megan and the narcotics.

When Allisyn felt comfortable Megan was fine, she left for the hospital to check on Conyers herself. She was reassured to see a police cruiser with two officers parked across the street from Megan's place.

At the hospital, she parked in the visitor garage and headed for the Emergency Department. She stopped at the triage desk to ask the receptionist where she could find Conyers.

"He's not here," she said gruffly. "He's been moved to the intermediate stay unit."

The place was chaotic. Stretchers in the halls because all the treatment bays were full, monitors beeping, patients moaning, relatives complaining, frazzled doctors barking orders, and hectic nurses rushing from one patient to the next. The waiting area appeared to be standing room only.

No wonder the receptionist is so ill-tempered.

"Ugh," Allisyn muttered under her breath as memories of her resident days rose intrusively from her subconscious. She shuddered to imagine having to go through it all again.

She didn't dare ask the unpleasant receptionist another question. Instead, she stopped who appeared to be a nurse's aide and asked where the intermediate stay unit was.

"Down the hall and to the left," he said, then turned and hurried over to a nurse irritably calling for him at a patient's bedside.

Allisyn rolled her eyes, shook her head, and hurried down the hall. When she arrived at the sign indicating the correct patient unit, she asked the receptionist for Conyers.

"Third bed on the left," she said pleasantly.

The ambiance was decidedly calmer and more civil.

When she reached the third stall, she shook the curtain and mockingly said "Knock-Knock."

"Yeah?" said Conyers with a weak voice.

He was partially sitting up in bed, his right arm in a sling and his shoulder heavily bandaged.

"Oh, hi there, Doctor," he said when he looked up. "I've been worrying about you and your niece. No one's been able to tell me if you were okay."

"You? Worried about me? Hell, you're the one who got shot."

He laughed. "Ow! That hurts," he said, gently touching his bandaged shoulder with the opposite hand.

"We're both fine. Phil Martinez took care of the bad guy. Apparently, a Nu-Genomix operative hell-bent on preventing disclosure of the missing research data."

"He's in custody?"

"Nah. In the morgue. Megan was pretty shaken up, but she's better now."

"Good." He winced as he shifted in bed to better face her. "Hold on. I need more of the happy juice." He pressed the call button for the nurse.

The nurse poked her head in almost immediately. "Yes, Detective?"

"Am I due for another pain shot?"

"Let me check."

She returned within a couple of minutes with a syringe. "Here you go," she said, and left after administering the medication.

"Hal, did you know about Martinez?" said Allisyn. "I mean, being an FBI agent?"

He closed his eyes momentarily, then looked up at her. "He was one of the agents present when I first met with the FBI after Clarissa Brenner's death. He didn't say much at all during the meeting. Agent Parkes did all the talking. He wasn't even introduced, as I recall. He just sat there listening. At the end of the meeting, he caught up with me before I left and explained how he was working on something that may be related to Nu-Genomix, and we should stay in touch with other." He paused, wincing again. "I didn't know until later that he was working undercover with you. He wanted to enlist my help in providing you with some protection. Seems he was concerned that you could be in danger, given all that was going on with Nu-Genomix. Sure was a good thing he was there today, though."

"Yeah. I didn't have a clue," she said. "I totally bought his story about being an investigative reporter. Seems his undercover work was investigating this Malaysian institute doing illicit human genetic engineering. The FBI's been working with international authorities, Interpol and the WHO. Turns out Nu-Genomix is connected to the operation, the Institute for Personal Enhancement. He got me involved because of my background in genomics and prior work with Paul Westin. He never even hinted he was law enforcement, just a reporter on the trail of a good story. I didn't know he was an FBI agent until today."

"Yeah, he wanted to keep that confidential. After all, that is the concept of undercover, right?"

"Yeah." She smirked. "He said the same thing when I went off on him about it. So what's the damage? To your arm?"

"Mainly muscle injury. They did a CT scan and a minor surgical exploration. Bullet went clear through, and they're pretty sure there's no nerve or blood vessel damage. I should be fine. Hurts like hell, though."

"Sorry."

"No worries. I'll be fine. Just glad the two of you are okay. And you can finally wrap this whole conspiracy thing up."

"Mm-hmm. I'll be getting the data to the FDA review team and it will stop any further review of their therapy. Phil will follow up with Interpol and the WHO. As far as the conspiracy part is concerned, the FBI's working on it now. I think . . ."

She noticed his eyelids drooping and his head nodding ever so slightly.

The nurse walked in. "How's he doing?"

Allisyn smiled. "Better, it seems."

"Yep," said the nurse. "Always does the trick."

"Guess I'll leave then. Let him know I'll check back with him later."

"Will do."

Allisyn dabbed the corners of her eyes with a tissue as she walked out.

On the way to her car she avoided passing through the Emergency Department with its grumpy receptionist.

CHAPTER

FIFTY

Julian Shawe had some good news to share with his investors. He decided to get them together for a status update on the gene therapy FDA application. Paul Westin joined him in the firm's boardroom. Jason Tinley was conspicuously absent. They hadn't been able to reach him for the last forty-eight hours.

"I'd like to welcome all of you again for another important update on the status of our gene therapy application process. We're approaching the end of the FDA's final review, and I'll let Dr. Westin fill you in on where we currently stand. Let me simply say you will be pleased indeed with what Paul has to say."

Westin remained seated. "Thank you, Julian. You may recall the FDA's Technical and Scientific Advisory Committee had previously recommended expedited review and possible approval of our therapy as a breakthrough treatment. We have now received notice our research data and some follow up information we were requested to supply has been favorably received by the actual CBER Review Committee, and our application approval is forthcoming. Our official letter of notification is in the process of being drafted."

Looking around at each other with nods of approval, everyone broke out in applause.

"Thank you. This has truly been a remarkable team effort by a large group of talented individuals. In view of this preliminary notification, we have initiated plans for an information and marketing campaign and also started reaching out to treatment centers around the country to notify them the therapy will be a viable option in the not too distant future. This is an exciting time for Nu-Genomix and, of course, the patients who will benefit from our innovative treatment. Now, I'll turn this back over to Julian."

"Thank you, Paul. I should point out there will be significant lead time before use of our therapy begins, and some time further before we will all realize any anticipated financial return, but I'm confident—"

He was interrupted by the ringing of the phone on a side table. Westin reached over to answer it, then nodded at Shawe and handed him the receiver.

Shawe listened for maybe thirty seconds, then hung up. He leaned over and whispered something to Westin, after which they both stood.

"Please excuse us for a few minutes," said Shawe. "We'll be right back."

There ensued light banter around the room as they waited for Shawe and Westin to return, mostly reverting back to everyone's delight at the news of the therapy's approval.

Shawe's assistant led them into a small, adjacent conference room and closed the door.

They both stood there, almost in shock.

"What the hell are you doing here?" demanded Westin.

Allisyn was sitting at a small conference table, tapping a flash drive on the table. "Have a seat, gentlemen. We'll be here awhile."

The two men looked at each other, confused. Shawe shrugged and sat. Westin followed suit.

"This flash drive in my hand holds all the evidence needed to prevent any further action on your application. Other than rejection, of course."

"You're bluffing," said Shawe.

Westin glared at her. "Let me see it."

"Not a chance."

"Where'd you get it?" asked Westin. "Probably a fake."

"Go ahead and believe that if you want. The CBER Review Committee already has a copy and verified it as authentic. The amount of negative research information you withheld from your application is astounding. Clear evidence of fraud."

"Really?" Westin scowled at her. He leaned back and folded his arms. "Guess you've been left out of the loop since your suspension. We've already received their approval letter."

Allisyn smiled at his smug response. "Approval? Huh. It was a mock letter from Dr. Francke. Intended to do exactly what it did. Keep you thinking all was well, until now. Your application is done. It's officially over."

Neither Shawe nor Westin said a word. They just stared at her.

"Now, let's talk about the Institute for Personal Enhancement."

Shawe glanced surreptitiously at Westin, then turned to Allisyn. "Excuse me?" he said.

"Hmm. Where should I start? Let's see, Nu-Genomix is part owner and operator of the clinic, you're on the board, Mr. Shawe, and you, Paul, you're a scientific adviser for the human genetic enhancement procedures they're performing. You do know those procedures are currently prohibited under the terms of an international ban, don't you?"

No answer. Shawe had a blank look on his face. Westin's stare was cold, his eyes narrowed, lips tight. Allisyn could almost feel his defiance.

"You're both complicit in the illegal performance of human genetic engineering, which has never been sanctioned by the international scientific community. Not to mention the numerous patient complications around the world because they're using your flawed gene technology under your guidance. The same form of complications you both knew existed from your research studies."

"You can't prove any of those accusations," declared Westin.

"Really? I believe authorities from the WHO, Interpol, and the FBI see things differently. And they want to speak with you both about it. They have evidence to the contrary, and a lot of questions for both of you."

She pulled out her phone and sent a quick text.

In a matter of seconds, an attractive but serious-looking woman entered alone. She wore a black pant suit over a white silk blouse.

"My name is Alondra Parkes," she said, displaying her FBI credentials. "I'm Deputy Special Agent in Charge for Science and Technology. Federal warrants have been issued for all information, files, data, electronic equipment and communications relative to the business of Nu-Genomix. Agents are currently initiating the warrants as we speak. Any attempts to destroy such material or otherwise impede the process is a federal crime."

She remained standing. "I also have warrants to take you both into custody for questioning with regard to your participation in a conspiracy to defraud the FDA. We have subpoenas to interview all Nu-Genomix employees and investors, and will be making arrangements for those interviews within the next few days. Agents are currently informing those individuals in the other room awaiting your return."

She walked over to the door and knocked twice. Two male agents entered and immediately took positions behind Shawe and Westin.

"It's been a pleasure speaking with you, gentlemen," Allisyn said as she put the flash drive in her pocket and left the room.

While Agent Parkes and Allisyn were finishing up with Shawe and Westin, three black Suburban vans pulled up to the main entrance of the research facility. A total of ten men and women exited the vehicles and headed for the front door. All wore lightweight, dark blue parkas with FBI emblazoned in large yellow letters on the back.

Upon entering the main entrance, a female agent went directly to the reception desk and introduced herself as she dutifully displayed her FBI credentials. She asked to speak with the most senior staff member present.

When the acting lab manager arrived, the agent handed him an envelope and gave him the same spiel about federal warrants Shawe and Westin had received, stressing any attempt to conceal or destroy all pertinent information would be a federal crime. "I also have a subpoena," she said, "granting us permission to interview, now or in the future, any employee or agent of the company. We'll begin the interviews right now with you and other members of management."

CHAPTER

FIFTY-ONE

"Hello, Allisyn," said Constance Vasquez tersely. She remained at her desk, eyes glaring at the visitor at her door. "I didn't expect to see you back until we had something to discuss. I thought I made it clear you were to have no further official contact until we sorted out your alarming situation."

Allisyn walked in and without any hesitation, sat down in the chair opposite the secretary's desk. "With the agency, you said. No further contact with the agency. You didn't say anything about you and me meeting to discuss the matter further. Although I must admit your assistant put up some resistance to letting me in. But I was pretty persistent, so please don't blame her."

Vasquez was unfazed by Allisyn's comments. "From what I remember when we last met, your behavior and actions—"

"I'm sorry," interrupted Allisyn, "Alleged behavior and actions. Alleged."

"Your . . . alleged behavior and actions regarding the Nu-Genomix gene therapy application are most disturbing, which I'm certain you understand. And the appropriate action was taken pending a thorough investigation."

"Really? Quite perplexing, considering how insistent you previously were that I intervene with the review committee to, let's say, encourage approval of the application. In fact, you were outright threatening as I recall."

Vasquez remained silent, glowering at Allisyn.

"So what has your investigation revealed?"

Shifting in her chair, Vasquez hesitated. "Surely you don't expect such an important inquiry to have been completed this quickly?"

"Of course not. I'm only looking for an update. Although no one has reached out to me as yet to obtain my version, which I find a little strange."

"Are you implying I'm not appropriately investigating these allegations?" blustered Vasquez. She sat up straight, back stiff, as she placed both hands—palms down—firmly on her desk. "How dare you come in here and make such an accusation!"

"I made no such accusation, Madam Secretary. I simply asked what you've determined thus far."

Vasquez huffed and leaned back. "I'm not at liberty to share anything with you at this point. As I said, my inquiry is not complete, but I haven't heard anything yet to contradict the allegations made against you."

"I see. And what have you learned about the missing research data? Data omitted from the Nu-Genomix application?"

"I'm sorry. I don't think I understand your question, since it was your allegation, and Mr. Shawe and Dr. Westin emphatically denied it. And as I recall, your accusation was based on hearsay, and you had no concrete evidence of such data."

"Really? Is it just a coincidence, then, my suspension was made public after I texted you I recently acquired the data?"

"I assumed it was a mere bluff. Besides, it had nothing to do with your suspension going public. We were getting inquiries from the media, and I, uh, needed to release a statement."

"How convenient." Allisyn smirked. "Oh, I almost forgot." She reached into her pocket and pulled out a USB flash drive, holding it up for Vasquez to see. "It seems such hard evidence of the data does exist after all. And I have it right here."

Vasquez was tightlipped and shook her head. "What . . . Where did you get that?"

"Where or how I got this is of no concern at the moment. What's important is it contains the full content of the data Nu-Genomix fraudulently omitted from their application. And it will successfully block approval of their application and discredit their bogus story I attempted to extort them."

Vasquez reached her hand out. "Let me see it."

"No way. You think I'm going to let this out of my possession and then have it disappear?"

"Why would I . . . Why would it disappear?"

"You really can't answer your own question, Constance? Or should I say . . . Camilla? Or possibly you would prefer Secretary Bartone.

"W-w-what are you talking about?"

"Camilla is your middle name, right? And Bartone is your maiden name. It's all here," she said, holding up an envelope.

Vasquez didn't respond. She sat very still, staring at Allisyn and appearing dumbfounded by what she was hearing.

"I guess you figured you could conceal your investment by putting it under a different name. And then further disguise it as a beneficiary of an obscure French investment trust whose only investment holding is Nu-Genomix stock shares. A healthy portion of the company, I might add."

Allisyn paused, expecting some kind of rebuttal. But none came.

Vasquez stared straight ahead as if looking right through Allisyn. She didn't say a word.

"What? You're not going to deny it?"

Vasquez leaned forward taking a menacing pose. "You're never going to prove any of this."

"Really? You've been wrong about me before. And if that's what you think now, you are again. My source is extremely reliable." Allisyn smiled at her own oblique reference to Phil Martinez.

Allisyn relaxed back in her chair. "First you tried to strong-arm me into making sure the gene therapy was approved because it would put Nu-Genomix on its way toward marketing it and generating profits, your ultimate goal. But not your only goal. It just so happens you've had a long-standing amorous relationship with Julian Shawe. In fact, he actually had a hand in getting you appointed HHS secretary."

Vasquez remained stone-faced.

"When I challenged Paul Westin about the concealed data and the treatment's harmful side effects, he and Shawe knew they had to neutralize me somehow. So the three of you concocted the bogus story I tried to trade approval of the application for a financial stake in the company. It gave you the premise to suspend me and ultimately discredit anything I might say. You had to protect your paramour and your investment."

Vasquez remained silent, her face beginning to redden.

"When I texted to let you know I finally had the data as evidence of their conspiracy to defraud the FDA, you announced my suspension and the presumptive reason to the public. But just to be certain I wouldn't cause any problems, you let Shawe know and he had his goon plan a more permanent arrangement for me. Which obviously didn't turn out well. Especially for the goon. Westin and your lover are having some very uncomfortable conversations with the FBI as we speak. And now it's your turn."

Allisyn stood and casually tossed an envelope on Vasquez's desk. "For your reading enjoyment." It was labeled "Camilla Bartone" and contained a copy of the information Martinez had procured for her. All the details of Vasquez's clandestine investment in Nu-Genomix, as well as her personal liaison with Shawe.

"I'll let myself out, Ms. Bartone. There's a gentleman waiting who has something else for you."

She walked over to the door and opened it. "You can come in now."

The gentleman stepped in, identified himself and flashed his FBI credentials. "I have a federal warrant for your detention for questioning regarding collusion in a conspiracy to defraud the federal government."

Allisyn left. Walking away, she tossed the flash drive into the air and caught it in her hand, making no attempt to suppress the smile on her face.

She had one more visit to make.

CHAPTER

FIFTY-TWO

Carlton Gradison read the text message from Allisyn on his cell. "Figured out Secretary Vasquez's interest in getting the Nu-Genomix gene therapy approved. Thought you'd want to know. When can we meet?"

He was puzzled. *Why is she texting me?* He really didn't want to engage with her but felt they'd better meet to learn exactly what she knew.

He texted her back to drop by his office late in the afternoon. He was planning to be working there into the early evening.

Allisyn arrived about five-thirty and was ushered into Gradison's office by his assistant.

"Welcome back, Doctor," said Gradison. "I'm anxious to hear what you've discovered about Secretary Vasquez. The political motive you were suspecting?"

"Don't think so," she said. "Turns out Constance Vasquez, under the name of Camilla Bartone, is a beneficiary of a French investment trust. It has only one investment. Shares in Nu-Genomix."

"Hmm. You think her attempt to pressure you into getting their application approved was motivated by her financial interest in the company? It would certainly make her a hefty profit if it went to market."

"Exactly. Except I refused to do her bidding to get the application approved. In the meantime, a would-be whistleblower and a dogged homicide detective's investigation of a deadly interaction between friends led to the discovery the gene therapy they were pushing had a serious flaw which resulted in a dangerous complication. And the information made its way to me."

"And with that information, you could prevent FDA approval of the therapy."

"Uh-huh."

"Ah, I see what you're getting at. She suspended you to get you out of the picture."

"You knew about my suspension?"

"Uh," he stammered, "I just heard about it on the news."

"Mm-hmm." Of course, the reason she suspended me was based on a false accusation in the first place. Although I guess she felt it was good enough, at least for the purpose of public consumption." She told him about Shawe and Westin's contrived extortion story and Vasquez's wild accusation Allisyn had lied to Congress about not having any intention to profit from any product under FDA review. "Unfortunately for them, I've since obtained a hard copy of the data they concealed. Their therapy, in its current form, will never get approved on my watch."

For the first time, he noticed the envelope she was holding. She was tapping it on her leg in an exaggerated manner. "Now, let's talk about your chief of staff and his role in all of this."

"I told you before. He was blackmailed by an operative of Nu-Genomix into applying pressure on you. They had evidence of his part in prior campaign contribution violations."

"Yes, I remember. But why was he killed?"

"Killed? The FBI concluded it was suicide, an intentional overdose. Because he was distraught over his legal situation after his attempt to extort you."

"That's what they thought before the autopsy. It so happens the post showed evidence of a struggle, bruises around his neck. Murder made to appear like a suicide."

"What? Why?"

"I'm disappointed, Senator. And you were doing so well up until now. He was killed to prevent him from cooperating with the police and FBI to save his own hide. Which would easily lead directly to the Nu-Genomix conspiracy to defraud the FDA with a falsified application and their blackmailing him to pressure me to approve it. Unfortunately for Mr. Krewe, his fate was sealed, just like the Nu-Genomix whistleblower, his sister and another lab worker, all with the aim of preventing the flaw in their therapy from being made public."

Allisyn sensed his rising anger, his tenseness, and saw the jutting of his jaw. His lips tightened as he glared at her. She could almost feel his eyes burning into her.

She broke the silence. "Now, should we discuss your own healthy investment in Nu-Genomix under your wife's maiden name, Marian Williams, by way of the same French foundation as Vasquez?"

He froze.

"I didn't think so. I do have one question, though. How did you bring yourself to throw your long-time friend and chief of staff under the bus?"

"W-w-what are you talking about?"

"Come on, Senator. You knew all along the Nu-Genomix operative was blackmailing him to put the pressure on me. It was probably your idea in the first place. Right?"

Silent, he stared at her with a menacing look.

"Of course it was. It kept you clean, and he took the fall. Harder than he could have expected, unfortunately."

Gradison stood and defiantly pushed his chair away. "This conversation is over. Any further questions can be directed to my lawyer."

"Seriously? Straight out of the movies?"

She took out her phone and fired off a one-word text. "Ready."

Within seconds, the door opened and his assistant let in a man in a dark suit.

He displayed his FBI credentials and identified himself as a special agent. He pocketed the badge and handed Gradison a document. "This is a signed warrant to take you into custody for questioning with regard to your complicity in a conspiracy to defraud the federal government."

Allisyn rose and walked out, but not before tossing the envelope on his desk. It was labeled "Williams" and contained a copy of the intel on Gradison that Martinez obtained for her.

CHAPTER

FIFTY-THREE

Allisyn requested an update meeting on the Nu-Genomix conspiracy investigation with Matthew Cleninger, Director of the FDA's Office of Criminal Investigation. The session was held at the Robert F. Kennedy Department of Justice Building on Pennsylvania Avenue. In addition to Allisyn and the Director, Deputy Special Agent Alondra Parkes and Phil Martinez were present to represent the FBI. Although not sure if he was up to it, Allisyn invited Hal Conyers, who had recently been released from the hospital.

"After all, you did get this entire process going," she told him.

"Are you kidding?" he said when she extended the invitation. "I wouldn't miss it for anything."

What a trooper, she thought.

Sure enough, he was right on time for the meeting. His arm was still in a sling, but the heavy bandaging was gone and it looked to Allisyn like his comfort level had definitely improved.

"Glad you could make it, Hal," she said "Feeling better?"

"Uh-huh. Down to one pain pill a day. Only to sleep at night."

"Great." She smiled at him. "You know, Hal, not sure if I ever properly thanked you for everything you did with Phil to keep me and Megan safe." Taking care to avoid his shoulder, she gave him a friendly hug. "I really had no idea."

He grinned. "Sure. No problem."

"Besides, it was you who got this whole investigation started by reaching out to Gardener about those three cases."

Director Cleninger spoke up and made introductions around the room. "We all know the basics of this investigation, so I don't think we need to rehash the details. My goal is just to provide an update on the status of the investigation."

He had a white board on which he diagrammed all the individuals involved in or otherwise affected by the conspiracy. It included the individuals who died—Gardener, Clarissa Brenner, Peroni, Seth Krewe—even Tinley.

Also depicted were the primary conspirators—Julian Shawe and Paul Westin—along with auxiliary participants, Constance Vasquez and Carlton Gradison.

Hal Conyers, Phil Martinez, and Allisyn herself were listed as participants in exposing the conspiracy and/or involved in the investigation. He emphasized Allisyn had been reinstated by the president to her position as FDA commissioner.

"Doctor McLoren," said Cleninger. "Can you update us on the status of the Nu-Genomix application process?"

"Certainly. Once I finally obtained a hard copy of the research data exposing the serious complication of their gene therapy, I turned it over to the CBER team reviewing the application. Their review concluded the data was authentic research material that had been omitted from their application documents. Based on the nature of the information, which demonstrated a disturbing complication of the treatment in both the animal models and human trials, they immediately suspended any further consideration of the therapy, denying approval for its use. It's indefinite at this point and not likely to be reversed."

Cleninger nodded. "From a legal perspective, the actions of the Nu-Genomix team show clear intent to defraud the FDA and meet the definition of a 'wrongful act' per our Application

Integrity Policy. Such conduct is treated as fraud perpetrated against the federal government." He paused, referring to some papers. "Special Agent Parkes?"

"Regarding the suspected conspirators," she said, "Julian Shawe and Paul Westin were initially detained for questioning and are being held with felony charges pending for conspiracy to defraud the government, as well as coercion, extortion, and blackmail in an attempt to have Dr. McLoren approve their application. Jason Tinley is deceased, of course, but considered responsible for the deaths of Gardener, Peroni, Brenner, and Krewe, as well as the attempted murder of Dr. McLoren and her niece, and assault with attempt to kill a federal agent and a local law enforcement officer. He was also guilty of blackmailing a nurse to falsely claim she observed Dr. McLoren's niece inappropriately accessing hospital opioids. Although Tinley was the perpetrator in each of those cases, Shawe and Westin are considered co-conspirators to commit murder as part of their roles in authorizing the cover-up. They most likely will be released with travel restrictions pending grand jury indictments. An injunction has been placed on the firm barring any further research related to their gene therapy, and all assets, monetary and otherwise, have been temporarily seized. Essentially, all activities of the firm have been ceased pending results of the full investigation. It's further expected Nu-Genomix will be subject to hefty monetary penalties from the government and numerous civil lawsuits for negligence causing significant harm by study patients and those treated at IPE. When all is said and done, the company is unlikely to survive as a viable research or other business entity."

Cleninger turned to Special Agent Martinez. "Could you please fill us in on your role in the FBI investigation?"

Martinez proceeded to explain the investigation in progress by the WHO and Interpol pertaining to the Institute for Personal Enhancement. The WHO considered IPE to be working outside of international norms. He explained he was initially working undercover on behalf of Interpol to identify U.S. investors in the facility. He then described how he came to team up with Allisyn, who subsequently identified documentation of the connection between Nu-Genomix and the Malaysian clinic. He concluded by saying the investigation by international authorities was ongoing. He deferred to Allisyn to describe the scientific link between the two organizations.

"Beyond the financial investment Nu-Genomix had in IPE," she said, "the practitioners at the Malaysian clinic were actually using the Nu-Genomix gene therapy technology to perform human enhancement procedures, even though the therapy had not yet been approved by the FDA for use. In fact, the flaw producing the complication Nu-Genomix withheld from their FDA application was exactly what was occurring repeatedly with IPE patients. The actual complication was different for each patient, however, depending on the specific genetic manipulation performed. The WHO continues to identify patients worldwide who were negligently affected."

Following Allisyn's comments, they wrapped up by agreeing to further meetings as necessary.

As Martinez and Allisyn walked out together, she gave him a flirtatious smile. "Up for a quick bite at Old Ebbitt's, then back to my place for a glass of wine?"

He smiled back. "I believe it would be a perfect end to the day."

CHAPTER

FIFTY-FOUR

After the meeting with the OCI and the other FBI agents, Allisyn and Martinez did as she suggested. They had a light dinner at Old Ebbitt's, then taxied over to her apartment, where they shared half a bottle of wine. And the rest of the night together. Sleep was sporadic.

The next morning, they showered and dressed. "I could make this a regular thing," said Allisyn with a glowing smile.

He laughed and pulled her close. Brushing her hair back, he kissed her forehead.

They kissed passionately, then she said, "Let's go to The Beanery for coffee and breakfast," It was the coffee shop down the block from her condo building where they first met after he had reached out to her as an investigative reporter.

It was a nice day and the shop was crowded, standing room only. They both ordered coffee, black, and a pastry.

The barista, a young man probably in his twenties seemed distracted as he handed them their order. As they turned to find a place to stand, they saw what had caught his attention. Everyone else in the café was intently looking up at the flat screen monitor on the wall.

"What's up?" Allisyn asked.

He just shrugged.

The monitor was tuned into a cable news station, and when the banner on the screen flashed *Breaking News*, they shared their suspicion of what was coming.

"Now for our lead story of the day. At a news conference within the last hour, the Department of Justice disclosed it has been conducting a sweeping investigation of a conspiracy to defraud the Food and Drug Administration. A biotech firm, Nu-Genomix, based in North Carolina, reportedly submitted fraudulent data in support of its application for approval to market its newly developed gene therapy for a certain form of heart disease. Information which showed a serious complication of the therapy resulting in at least three deaths of clinical trial patients was withheld from the FDA.

"The conspiracy also involved a scheme of coercion and blackmail to gain approval of their flawed product and involved the willing participation of Health and Human Services Secretary Constance Vasquez, who allegedly has a significant financial interest in Nu-Genomix. Vasquez has been removed from her cabinet position by the president. Also implicated as an investor was Senator Carlton Gradison, who was purported to be his party's leading candidate for president. He has withdrawn his name from consideration and resigned his Senate seat."

A number of gasps and expressions of shock could be heard from some of the patrons.

"In a written statement, FDA Commissioner Dr. Allisyn McLoren noted review of the product has been halted indefinitely."

Allisyn cringed and was silently relieved the report was not accompanied by her photo. Nevertheless, she slunk to the back of the room adjacent to the door. Martinez moved back with her, gently placing his arm around her waist.

"Dr. McLoren stressed the FDA remains committed to the development of innovative forms of treatment supported by valid research data which safely provide a proven benefit for patients."

"Yeah, right," one patron uttered aloud. "Proactive government oversight for ya."

Several other patrons laughed. Allisyn closed her eyes for a moment and shook her head as the news report continued.

"In a prepared statement at this morning's press conference, FBI Lead Investigator Deputy Special Agent for Science and Technology Alondra Parkes confirmed several deaths may be related to attempts at a cover-up, including Gradison's chief of staff.

"Attorney General Amanda Hesterton stated this represents an unprecedented conspiracy to defraud the U.S. Government, endangering the integrity of the FDA and the safety of the American public."

More murmurs and comments of concern and distrust of government could be heard among the patrons.

"In a related development, a medical clinic located in Kuala Lumpur, Malaysia, with ties to China as well as Nu-Genomix, has been identified as performing procedures described as non-disease-related elective genetic engineering using the flawed Nu-Genomix technique for numerous individuals from multiple countries, many of whom have experienced complications. The FDA is collaborating with the World Health Organization to further investigate the connection between the Institute, China, and Nu-Genomix.

Allisyn and Martinez tossed their empty coffee cups into a trash receptacle and turned to leave for the short walk back to her condo.

"It's too early for wine," she said as they walked hand in hand.

"I know. But that's not what I had in mind."

She smiled, and they picked up their pace.

CHAPTER

FIFTY-FIVE

"This committee is now in session." Senator Emmit Prentiss banged the gavel, convening the special meeting of the Senate HELP Committee. As a senior member of the committee, Prentiss assumed the chairman position when Carlton Gradison stepped down and relinquished his senate seat under pressure from his party.

After exposing the Nu-Genomix conspiracy, as well as its illicit and dangerous collaboration with the Chinese at the Institute for Personal Enhancement, Allisyn was once again appearing before the Senate committee. Prior to the start of the hearing, she browsed the room's crowded gallery, taking special note of three participants sitting together —Phil Martinez, Hal Conyers, and Megan.

"I'd like to welcome Dr. McLoren and express our appreciation for her meeting with us today," said Senator Prentiss. "Dr. McLoren?"

"Thank you for the invitation to present my perspective on the various issues which have come to light as a result of this recently thwarted conspiracy to defraud the FDA. I especially want to thank Chairman Prentiss for honoring my request this be an open, public hearing. It is extremely important for everyone, not just our government representatives, to recognize this conspiracy is not only a series of criminal acts which have been committed. It also represents scientific deception of the highest degree. The

FDA is charged with evaluating such a therapy for effectiveness and safety. Withholding evidence of a known serious complication of the therapy is not only fraud perpetrated against the FDA. It is, in fact, fraud perpetrated against the American public itself, demonstrating a blatant disregard for the potential threat it posed for patients unaware of their flawed medical treatment."

She paused to take a sip of water before continuing.

"On another level, however, the actual issues at the core of the legitimate use of gene therapy, its promise and its perils, must be carefully considered by the scientific community. The highly questionable practice of human genetic engineering, such as that performed at the Institute for Personal Enhancement, lacked international endorsement. In the face of a current ban and with disregard for patient safety, such practice must be addressed by both the scientific community and society as a whole.

"I will not address the specific details of the conspiracy here today. I'm sure members of the committee are familiar with them by now, as they have been clearly enumerated in the Justice Department's indictment documents and public statements. For my part, this episode of scientific deception clearly justifies the agency's insistence on a measured and thorough process in evaluating any new drug or medical therapeutic product before approval for market availability. As a central component of such a process, data integrity is paramount in the evaluation process. When it breaks down, whether inadvertently or intentionally, as in this case, the evaluation of what is being tested itself becomes both imprecise and unreliable.

"The FDA review and evaluation process is deliberate to ensure the public of a therapeutic's efficacy and safety, not because of inefficiency or to intentionally delay any worthy treatment. The current case in question was clearly intended to circumvent this process.

"Going forward, we must not appease those who decry over-regulation and instead resist calls to compromise our process in the name of making innovative and cutting edge therapies available to the public hastily at any cost.

"Gene therapy is an exciting scientific innovation with the medical possibility to help many patients with difficult or impossible to treat diseases of genetic origin. This is intricate and complex business, however, and complications can occur under the best of circumstances. Nevertheless, let us not be foolish and, as the saying goes, throw the baby out with the bath water. Admittedly, an ironic aphorism given the topic."

"Like nuclear power and many other great accomplishments of modern science, gene therapy holds incredible potential for mankind but also creates the opportunity for misuse, accidental at best, intentional for illegitimate or wrongful purposes at worst. For this, we must remain forever vigilant and unremitting in demanding the highest degree of oversight.

"The challenging technical aspects related to the successful use of gene therapy aside, we cannot ignore the questions we as a society must address in routinely utilizing this medical technology. Ethical, moral, even legal, social, and economic questions. Gene therapy for the treatment of disease when appropriate is one thing. But using the technology to alter our DNA for the sole purpose of enhancing any human trait or performance, physical, intellectual, or other, is something altogether different."

She took another sip of water. Scanning the committee membership, she sensed her words were being received with the greatest level of gravity.

"The final piece of this scandal, which has international ramifications, is what we learned about the Institute for Personal Enhancement, initially thought to be the sole doing of the Chinese. Unfortunately, Nu-Genomix surreptitiously conspired with them as a partner in performing genetic engineering using their own flawed synthetic gene technology. These enhancement procedures were performed on individuals from many countries, ours included. With the cooperation of the WHO, we are only now learning the extent to which this has occurred, with the number of patients so treated growing daily. Unfortunately, the number of those identified with serious complications as a side effect is also growing. This is clearly a tragedy of global proportions." She paused, lips pursed while nodding. "Yes, Nu-Genomix is no longer an active participant since the cessation of its operations. And although the Malaysian government has rightly revoked the ability for IPE to perform such procedures, we must ensure the practice does not continue at alternate venues. Fortunately, international pressure is growing via numerous channels to prevent any further use of this flawed genetic enhancement technique.

"In the end, all this duplicitous and fraudulent behavior was driven by one simple motivation—the desire for corporate and individual profits. What started out as a potentially legitimate medical venture devolved into one seeking inordinate financial gain. Such is the fate of legitimate scientific research when it becomes subservient to corporate greed and power. Let us learn a lesson and be ever wary of the subjugation of science, research, and the treatment of disease to the less noble goal of financial gain. And let us never forget the primary dictum of the medical profession as defined by the Hippocratic Oath. First, do no harm."

She closed the folder holding her notes and looked up at the panel of senators, hesitating briefly before continuing.

"Finally, let me close with this. In applying genetic manipulation technology to humans, we must reflect on how we differentiate between needed therapy and elective enhancement, otherwise referred to as human genetic engineering. When does a genetic intervention intended to cure a condition become over time something to enhance an individual's normal attributes? And through elective genetic enhancement, are we actually changing what we consider to be normal in the first place? Does genetic enhancement provide an unfair advantage, whether it be in academics, sports, or competition for resources? How do we rationalize financial disparities which allow for some individuals to afford such elective enhancement and others not? Or is this no different than any other discretionary acquisition based on affordability? If you're wondering, I'm not here to provide answers to these questions. Instead, my message is to urge a thoughtful discussion among the best and brightest minds in the fields of science and medicine, ethics, and law, even religion, to address these questions. And many others, more complex, before we proceed with wholesale use of this technology. And such discussions should include the public's perspective.

"In summary, all these questions speak to the overall concept of social equality. Having the capability to do something so dramatic does not necessarily give us the absolute license to do it."

"This concludes my statement."

No questions were posed from committee members. There was, however, a brief period of subdued but widespread applause.

She couldn't see them, but Martinez, Conyers, and Megan were nodding and beaming in approval.

EPILOGUE

The Nu-Genomix conspiracy had become a top story that wouldn't go away in all manner of news outlets. There was no shortage of public appetite for conjecture and vilification of government oversight. An unseemly and potentially dangerous outcome was successfully averted, although such reality seemed to be less popular in the court of public opinion.

Allisyn returned to the FDA full-time as commissioner at the order of the president, since Vasquez had been dismissed. Her statement to the Senate HELP Committee was widely acclaimed in all circles—research, medical, legal, and bio-ethical— and lauded as a seminal call to action to evaluate the future of elective human genetic manipulation.

Megan slowly returned to her normal state of emotions, although for a while she had recurring nightmares related to her harrowing experience with Tinley. The manufactured accusation of her misappropriating hospital opioids was discredited and dismissed. In the end, the rigors of a medical residency provided little time and residual energy for her to dwell on the event. On the positive side, she and Allisyn spoke about the future more frequently than ever. She had decided to proceed with pursuing a research-based fellowship in infectious disease, hoping to go on to a career in public health.

Hal Conyers was recovering nicely. His wound had healed and his rehab was progressing smoothly. On one occasion, he traveled to North Carolina with his wife to put flowers on Bryce Gardener's grave. It seemed to provide some degree of closure for him, and he was finally able to put to rest his obsession with the terrible Cliffden death, as well as the other two. He still thought occasionally about how unlikely it was they led to exposing the Nu-Genomix conspiracy.

Allisyn's newfound relationship with Martinez continued unabated, although neither broached the subject of a more permanent arrangement.

One Saturday evening, they were having dinner at DaNino's, her favorite Italian restaurant on M Street in Georgetown. It reminded her of the kind of place she preferred to eat while in Rome. Simple white tablecloths—not tacky white and red checkered plastic—and waiters who actually spoke Italian. Great house Chianti served in open carafes and the absolute best Spaghetti Cacio e Pepe this side of Tuscany.

Their discussion covered a number of topics over dinner, mostly related to favorite pastimes and hobbies, but none regarding the ongoing investigation. When they finished eating, Martinez called the waitress over and ordered two cappuccinos.

"Wait," said Allisyn. "Make it two espressos."

The waitress turned and walked away.

"What's with that?" he said.

"Don't you know cappuccino is never consumed after the morning? At least in Italy?"

"Really? So why did you offer to make cappuccino the first time you invited me up to your place, huh? It was late afternoon, early evening."

She grinned. "I thought if I said wine, at least before we got there, I'd scare you off."

"Yeah, right." He grinned back.

When they finished their coffees, she waved the waitress over and ordered two glasses of Campari.

"Now what?" he said.

"You've never heard of it?"

"Uh-uh."

"It's an Italian bitter aperitif. You'll like it once you get used to it."

When the waitress returned, they clinked their glasses and sipped.

He winced just a bit, then nodded. "Interesting. Quite good, actually." He took another sip. "I must say I've learned a good bit from you tonight."

"Be patient." She winked. "The night is young."

Almost choking on his drink, he cleared his throat and waved the waitress over for the check. "Then let's not waste any time."

They caught a cab and when they got to her condo, she opened a fresh bottle of Chianti. They sat together on the couch, once again enjoying the view of the waterfront out the window while discussing the outcome of the investigation. Some mellow Wynton Marsalis was softly playing in the background.

"What's the latest word from the DOJ?" she asked.

"You didn't hear it from me, but the Grand Jury's returning indictments for Shawe and Westin for conspiracy to defraud the government and commit murder. Announcement is planned for tomorrow."

"What about Gradison and Vasquez?"

"Nothing definite yet. Although Vasquez is gone as a result of her clandestine and inappropriate investment in IPE, she's still subject to criminal charges for extortion for trying to coerce you into approving their application by threatening your career and reputation. Something Gradison doesn't have to worry about— yet. If they can prove he was part of the scheme to blackmail Krewe into pressuring you, that's a different story and may result in criminal charges for him as well. After being forced by his party to vacate his Senate seat, I would guess his political future is pretty much nonexistent."

They were both silent for a short spell as they sipped their wine.

"Have you been in contact with the WHO?" asked Martinez.

"As a matter of fact, they've reached out to me for help in identifying the specific genetic defects resulting in the complications showing up so far in patients who underwent the enhancement procedure. They've actually identified quite a significant number of patients showing side effects. The whole process is pretty complicated. Obviously, the gene affected depends on which characteristic was being targeted for enhancement, which in turn will determine what complication might follow. Sort of like a genetic jigsaw puzzle. Speaking of which, any news on how the Edgers girl and Amanda Leyfferts are doing?"

"Felicity Edgers had surgery to remove the muscle tumor. Last I heard she was doing well."

"For now. I suspect she unfortunately may need more treatment."

Martinez shook his head. "As for Leyfferts, she must be fine. She's back on her TV show and pretty active otherwise, from what my sources tell me."

Allisyn smiled. "Your sources, eh? Like Interpol?"

"Yeah. And others."

There was another silence between them before Martinez spoke.

"And you, Allisyn? How does it feel getting back on the job?"

"Okay."

He frowned. "Just okay?"

"I mean, the staff have been great and all. Very supportive, in fact. Nobody believed Vasquez's ridiculous story anyway."

"So? What else?"

"It's the politics. I just have no appetite for it. I do my job the best I can and hope it all works out."

"Not a bad approach, actually. Although it is Washington after all. Just roll with it. He gently brushed a wisp of hair off her forehead. "Given you were so quickly reinstated, you're obviously as well regarded as you've always been."

"I guess."

"But?"

"Actually, the president called me for a meeting. He wants me to consider the HHS secretary position in his Cabinet."

Martinez sat up straight, eyes wide. "Fantastic! Why haven't you told me sooner?"

"Just happened. Besides, not sure I want it. Like I said, politics."

"Come on, Allisyn. Get serious. Do you know how much you could influence this whole genetic enhancement conversation by holding such a position? Not to mention health care in general. This is perfect for you."

"I don't know. I'm a researcher, not a demagogue."

He turned toward her and looked deeply into her eyes. "A pretty narrow view of the world, I'd say. You have so much to offer. You absolutely must accept the appointment."

"We'll see." She just stared out the window, trance-like, deep in thought. She looked down at the wine glass in her hand briefly, then back up at him "There's something I need to share with you, Phil. I didn't tell you the entire story when I said I was engaged but the relationship fell apart. It wasn't just the distance. I had an affair . . . with Paul Westin while we worked together in Rome. A brief one. While I was engaged to Jordan. I had an affair, Phil. It was only a dalliance and meant nothing. Just a distraction from the pressure of the research we were doing. When I returned, I could never bring myself to tell Jordan. The guilt tormented me constantly, and I came to doubt whether I could ever be trusted. Not just in a relationship, but anything. And little by little, it destroyed what we had. Ironic, isn't it? He never knew, but it tore us apart."

Martinez put his hand on hers. "It's okay, Allisyn. It happens. It's not the end of—"

"Don't you see?" She had a pained expression on her face. "I've fallen in love with you, Phil. It's unlike any other feeling

I've ever had. But I don't trust myself, my feelings, my emotions. I second guess everything. Like with the president. I—"

"Stop, Allisyn. You can't go on like this. It was a momentary lapse. Nothing more. It can happen to anybody, anytime."

She looked at him. "That's what Megan said."

"Smart woman, that Megan." He paused briefly. "And for what it's worth, I've fallen in love with you as well. Deeply. Deeper than I would have ever imagined possible. Your beauty, your strength, your kindness and concern for others, your commitment to what you do and believe in. I see it all when you talk with Megan. All of it." He turned toward her and kissed her passionately.

"I won't let you torment yourself any longer, Allisyn. I've been there myself, and I don't ever want to go back."

They embraced deeply.

He pulled away and looked at her. "I think this is the start—"

"No. Don't say anymore. That's my favorite movie."

They both laughed.

And she finally knew, once again, what it was like to trust herself.

Acknowledgments

As in all creative endeavors, scientific or literary, it all begins with an idea. My initial idea, to write a novel based on my professional background, was inspired by a medical fiction writing conference where I was fortunate to meet and learn from two icons in the genre, Tess Gerritsen and the late Michael Palmer.

My story idea, the basis for WRONGFUL ACTS, came shortly thereafter, but mostly remained dormant due to professional and family responsibilities. Until I retired several years ago.

To be successful, however, any such endeavor requires the encouragement and support of others to succeed, and I would like to thank the following.

The library staff of the hospital where I worked who provided the extensive literature search on gene therapy and human genetic engineering which is the scientific basis for Wrongful Acts.

I also want to give a huge shout out to my developmental editor, Jeff Ayres, who provided numerous recommendations to improve my original manuscript, and Jon Land, established author whom I met at ThrillerFest and recommended Jeff to me. Both provided the needed encouragement to keep me going. And Susan Sutphin, whose final edit helped me put the finishing touches on the manuscript.

For those who provided a beta read of my early manuscript, Sue DiTommaso and Cathy Kramp, thanks for taking the time and providing honest feedback that allowed me to re-think many aspects of that original version.

To my good friend Greg Cannizzaro, who created an exceptional design for my logo, capturing my background as a physician and current aspiration for writing, a big thanks and welcome to the beach, paesano!

To the staff of eBook Launch, Dane and John, for their amazing work in designing the cover for WRONGFUL ACTS and the interior formatting, thanks for a great job.

Finally, but perhaps most important, is the support of my family. From the continued prodding of my three children—Andrew, Greg, and Nicole—over the years to "just write your book!" to the invaluable advice and insight into editing and publishing Nicole provided along the way.

And in the spirit of saving the best for last, is the endearing and endless support and encouragement of my wife, Alexis, along with her incredible patience in listening to all my self-doubts and frustrations.

Thanks to all of you. I couldn't have done it without you!

ABOUT THE AUTHOR

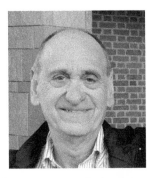

Anthony "Tony" Sclama is a retired physician who practiced Urology for twenty-two years and served as a hospital executive for eleven years in Baltimore, Maryland. A Rhode Island native, he graduated from Georgetown University and received his MD degree from the University of Maryland School of Medicine, where he completed his residency in Urologic Surgery. He also holds a Master's degree in Business-Healthcare Management from the Johns Hopkins University School of Continuing Studies.

He has three adult children and currently resides in Bethany Beach, Delaware with his wife, Alexis.

To learn more about Tony and his writing go to www.tonysclama.com

CPSIA information can be obtained
at www.ICGtesting.com
Printed in the USA
LVHW030106191121
703740LV00010B/961